Prepping Your Family for an Emergency

SIMPLE STEPS TO STAYING SAFE DURING A DISASTER.

Suzanne Lowe

Suzanne Lowe/Silvergum Publishing

www.suzanneloweauthor.com

www.silvergumpublishing.com

Cover Shutterstock/Silvergum Publishing

Prepping your home for an emergency/Suzanne Lowe —1st ed.

ISBN 9780648904915

A catalogue record for this work is available from the National Library of Australia

*To my family, Steve, Tahlia and
Emilie.*

*"When we have each other, we have
everything."*

*Hope for the best but prepare
for the worst.*

−Prepper mantra

Contents

Introduction

There are many books on preparing or prepping for a long-term worldwide disaster such as an EMP blast, nuclear war, or meteor strike. ***Prepping your family for an emergency*** is not that type of book, nor is it a Bear Grylls wilderness survival guide. ***Prepping your family for an emergency*** is a book for the average family and focuses on what you need to do in a short-term crisis to keep your family safe and fed in your own home. This includes an event such as an extended power outage, pandemic, flood, bushfire, cyclone, hurricane, or any other event that forces your family into self-isolation, lockdown, or short term "bunking in."

In 2017 Hurricane Katrina caused widespread damage and loss throughout New Orleans, in 2019 Typhoon Odai killed over 900 people in Africa, and in early 2020 bushfires ravaged Australia and an unexpected pandemic hit the world. Movie theatres, gyms, schools, restaurants, and many other services we take for granted were suddenly shut down. Many countries saw panic buying of goods such as hand sanitizer, toilet paper, rice, pasta, and medical supplies. Shelves were left bare and restrictions were placed on purchases.

Families were forced to quarantine inside their homes, international travel was placed on hold and countries were placed in lockdown as Governments tried to stem the spread of infection.

Many people were unprepared for these disasters and unsure what they needed to keep their homes and families safe. They had to rely on authorities for help and this help was not always immediately available.

Prepping your family for an emergency will provide you with a guideline of what you will need if your family finds themselves confined to home whether it be from a man-made disaster or event such as a prolonged power outage or a natural disaster such as a flood or severe storm.

Easy recipes including hand sanitizer, disinfectant and simple to prepare meals are included at the back of the book, using food and items from your pantry.

Stay safe and remember the prepper's motto, *hope for the best but prepare for the worst!*

Suzanne Lowe

Chapter One

What do you need for short-term isolation?

If your family must go into quarantine, or you want to be prepared in case of a lockdown, power failure or natural disaster, there are some things you can easily do without going on a wild spending spree. Some of the foods and items you may already have in your home.

Remember, you can't prepare for every scenario. Instead prepare for what you see as the greatest threat to your family.

All foods and items suggested can be adjusted to suit your own family's tastes and size.

Let's start with a few handy tips:

Purchase what your family likes to eat, and you feel comfortable preparing. If you purchase twenty tins of tomatoes just because they are on sale, however, you hate tomatoes they will only take up space in your home and be a waste of your money.

Be prepared to substitute. You may not have the exact ingredients for a particular meal you want to make, and you won't be able to *pop to the shops* to buy it. Instead substitute.
For example, substitute rice instead of pasta or spaghetti, use different beans, vegetables, herbs, and spices. Don't be afraid to get creative.

Freeze leftovers. When cooking meals for your family, prepare extra and freeze the leftovers. For example, meat or vegetable sauce for pasta, soups, casseroles, and stews all freeze well. Place the leftovers in Ziplock bags and label with the date and contents using a permanent marker. Remove the air from the bags before sealing and lay flat in your freezer. Storing food in smaller serves helps it freeze quickly and means you can defrost only what you need.

Freeze chopped fruit and vegetables. When fresh fruits and vegetables are not available, or you are not able to get to the store, frozen fruit and vegetables are a great alternative for use in cooking.

However, it should be noted that not all fruit and vegetables freeze well, for example, lettuce will become soggy after being frozen. For more information and tips on which vegetables and fruits freeze well, see the chapter *How to freeze fruits and vegetables.*

Freeze plastic bags or containers of water. These can be used in a cooler/esky to help keep food cold, or for drinking water once thawed. They are also useful for injuries where an icepack is required or to cool the body during hot weather. Simply wrap the frozen water bag in a light cloth before placing on the skin.

Have alternate cooking methods available. When the power goes out, or you are unable to access your usual cooking supplies it is important to have an alternative, safe method available. See the chapter *Cooking in a disaster* for examples of alternate cooking methods you can use.

Rotate your food supplies. To ensure your food stays fresh and you are not stuck with a whole lot of food past it's use by date, get into the habit of rotating the food in your pantry, freezer and storage areas. Check your food regularly. When any food supplies are coming close to their use by date, use those first and replace with new stock. Whenever you purchase food, remember, *newest to the back, oldest to the front.*

Have enough non-perishable food for 3-4 weeks. You will need enough food supplies such as tinned, packaged, dried and preserved food to provide your family with three meals per day for 3-4 weeks.

Don't forget the furry and feathered members of your household. You will also need to have enough food for any pets you have in the house as well.

Have an emergency cash supply. This doesn't need to be a large amount of money; however, it is always useful in case you cannot get to the bank, the ATMs are not available, or you need a ready source of money and cannot leave your home.

Have a family emergency plan. Everyone in your family including children should know what to do in case of emergencies. For example, who is picking the children up from school?
Do the older children, teenagers and young adults in your family make their own way back home or will you be picking them up? See the chapter *Making a plan of Action* for further advice.

Don't spend too much money on things you won't use. Unless you are prepping for a doomsday scenario where your family must leave you home and "bug out" to another location you are not likely to need a GPS tracker or satellite phone. There are a multitude of survivalist items available to purchase, some of them expensive. If you don't think your family will need them, save your money and purchase items you can use at home such as extra batteries or a camp stove.

Have an adequate water supply.
Ideally have a drinkable water supply for all members of your family including pets for at least three days. See the chapter on *How much water do I need?* for further advice.

Have an emergency and first aid kit in your home.
Everyone in the family should know where these are located in your house. The appendices at the end of the book give you examples of first aid and family emergency kits.

Have enough of your prescription medicine.
Make sure you have enough supplies of your usual prescription medicines to last at least a month. During and after an emergency such as a flood, cyclone, or hurricane for example, it may take time for pharmacies to restock their supplies. Especially if roads and rail lines are closed.

Chapter Two

Make a Plan of Action

To help your family stay safe, you should have a *family plan of action*. Everyone in the household needs to be aware of this action plan. You can also include other family members such as grandparents and friends if you wish.

For example, your action plan could include:

Make a list of medical and emergency numbers.

Keep this list in an easily accessible location for all family members to access if needed. The refrigerator or a pin-up board are good places. Your list can also include school and work numbers.

Have a hard copy of your contacts.

Like the medical and emergency numbers it is also a good idea to have a hard copy of your family and friend's contact numbers somewhere accessible.

Who is most at risk in your family?

For example, older people, pregnant women, and people with underlying health risks such as asthma or diabetes or compromised immune systems may be more at risk.

Speak to your General Practitioner about what extra assistance they might need and how you can minimize any infection. For example, during a pandemic, those at a higher risk may need to eat separately from the family and maintain a distance of 2 meters from other household members.

Where can you isolate if a family member becomes sick or infected?

Identify a room/s you can use to isolate one or more of your family members if they become sick/infected. This area will need to be cleaned regularly to help stop the spread of infection to other family members.

If you have more than one bathroom or toilet in your home, dedicate one of the bathrooms/toilets to the sick members of the family.

Who is picking up the kids?

Emergencies don't always happen when everyone is together and at home. You should have a pre-agreed plan on who will pick up the children from school/day-care/after school activities in case of a disaster such as an impending cyclone? Do older children and teenagers in the family need to make their own way home or will you come and pick them up?

Are you staying in your home or relocating/bugging out?

Depending upon the particular emergency you are experiencing and its severity you may need to consider whether it is safer to stay in your home or leave for a more secure location. If you decide to leave, make sure you know in advance where you are travelling to and alternate routes to get there.

Chapter Three

Prepare your home for lockdown or isolation.

Cleaning and sanitizing

Get into the habit of washing your hands regularly with soap and water for 20-minutes, especially when you have been out of the house (for example, at work or buying food/ petrol etc. or at the park with your children).

Regularly clean door handles and cupboard knobs, refrigerator handles, oven and microwave doors, computer keyboard and mouse, and television remote controls. These items would be regularly touched by household members.

Family members working away from the home before a lockdown is enforced (for example, health care workers and grocery store attendants) should have a designated area where they can remove shoes and coats when returning home. Spray these with a disinfectant. These family members should also wash their hands thoroughly or use hand sanitizer before coming into contact with other family members.

Purchase enough food and medical supplies for at least three weeks of isolation. (See the Appendices on food and medical supplies for suggestions on what you might need).

Go Local

Plan to use smaller, local supermarkets, ATMs, petrol/gas stations and pharmacies as they will have less people using them as opposed to the larger centres. Make sure you wash your hands thoroughly or use hand sanitizer after using petrol/gas pumps, ATMS, cash machines, touch screens, elevator buttons, shopping trolly handles or escalator handrails.

Limit the number of visitors coming to your home.

Keep the number of people coming into your home who are not your immediate family to a minimum. The fewer number of people you encounter the risk of becoming infected decreases. Many people will not show outward signs of infection until many days or even weeks after they are contagious.

Skip fast food/uber eats particularly from chain restaurants where a lot of people might be visiting.

Sanitize any deliveries.

Before bringing any deliveries including letters and parcels into your home, they should be sanitized or left for three hours before handling. Wipe or spray with disinfectant or use gloves and wash your hands with soap and water afterwards.

Chapter Four

Preventing Infection

Once a virus has started to spread throughout the community and become a pandemic, the chances of infection increase.

To decrease your risk of infection the Centre of Disease Control recommends you follow these rules.

Keep your distance.

Stay 1.5 to 2 metres away from other people and try to keep away from crowed areas unless absolutely necessary.

Sanitize your hands.

Use soap and water to lather and wash your hands for at least 20 minutes, especially if you have been outside your home or in contact with other people. Don't forget to wash between your fingers.

Alcohol based hand sanitizer can also be used.

Stay Hydrated.

Drink plenty of warm fluids to keep your body hydrated and to help flush any contaminants from your throat into your stomach. Here your stomach acids can help neutralize them.

Sneeze and cough into a tissue.

Try and keep germs away from other people by sneezing or coughing into a tissue and throwing the tissue away. Alternatively sneeze or cough into the crook of your arm. If you cough/sneeze into your hands and then touch something, germs are more easily spread.

Wear a face mask.

If you are infected or suspect you may be infected, wear a face mask to prevent the spread of germs to other people, particularly members of your household as they will be in close contact with you.

Seek Medical advice.

If you are ill or have reason to believe you are infected, seek medical advice and be prepared to self-isolate.

Washing.

Wash clothes, shower, and wash hair regularly especially after leaving your home to go the supermarket or other areas where many people have been. *Centre of Disease Control. www.cdc.gov*

Chapter Five

How to sanitize your food

Fruits and vegetables

Wash fresh produce (fruits and vegetables) in warm soapy water to remove any contaminants, then rinse in fresh running water. Viruses can remain on surfaces for 3 days.

Fill a sink with hot water and some dish washing detergent.
Fill a 2nd sink, a large bowl, or bucket with cold water. Separate leaves for lettuce etc. for easy access to clean.

Plunge your fruit and vegetables into the soapy water. Swish it around and scrub if necessary. Work in small batches to reduce the time spent in the water (they don't need to soak).

Then, wash under cold running water to rinse off the soap or plunge into your bowl/bucket of cold water. Dry on a dish rack or similar to drain.
Store as you ordinarily do.

Meat, fish, seafood don't need to be sanitized as they are going to be cooked (usually over a high heat).

Food in cans, jars and packets usually don't need to be sanitized, however if you want to be extra cautious these can be stored separately from your other food for three days before adding to your pantry.

For vulnerable people (elderly and people with a low immunity)

For the elderly and people with a lower immunity, every item that enters the kitchen needs to be sanitized or separated for three days (e.g., in a box, separate fridge) before being put in the pantry/fridge.

This includes:

bottles and jars of sauces, spreads

cans of vegetables

packets of noodles, dried beans, frozen vegetables

bottles of fruit juice, drinks

packets/bottles of dried herbs

meat (wash the outside packaging)

products in paper bags. These can be wiped with disinfectant wipes or sprayed and wiped.

toiletry products such as toothpaste, face wash, shaving cream and any other personal hygiene items, particularly those for the face, eyes, and mouth.

Chapter Six

Ten tips to make life in isolation easier.

Suddenly having to live in isolation when you are used to being able to go out and do whatever you like, whenever you want can be a challenge. Follow these 10 tips to make the experience easier.

1. Focus on the positives. You're in the comfort of your own home. You get to spend quality time with your family. You can do many of the things you never usually have time for!

2. Schedule a much-needed job to do each day.

3. Have a family board game night.

4. Open your windows each day and let the fresh air in.

5. Spend some time outside each day even it is only on your balcony or front porch. Vitamin D is good for your health and immunity.

6. Stay in touch with your relatives and friends by Skype, Messenger, Facetime etc. Being able to see other people is a boost to your mental health.

7. Keep a diary of your thoughts and what you did during the day. You might find it interesting to look back on your experience in years to come.

8. Don't spend all your time on the computer or watching TV. Be productive. Do things you've been wanting to do.

9. Do some exercise even if it's only stretching or walking around your apartment or backyard. There are also plenty of exercise programs on YouTube.

10. Don't be afraid to tell your family, friends or housemates that you need some space for a couple of hours. It's not easy to *live on top* of each other and having time to yourself is important. If you find yourself getting frustrated or angry at your situation or your housemates, take a break and do something by yourself.

Chapter Seven

Food Supplies

If you've ever seen the empty food shelves in supermarkets after a *run*-on food supplies, you'll know that having your own *emergency pantry* at home is a good idea.

Most stores do not carry a lot of extra stock because of the risk of spoilage, costs, and space. This is especially true for smaller stores. This means that if deliveries to the stores are disrupted because of a disaster then, once the stock on the shelves are bought, they won't be replenished until new deliveries can be made and this could be weeks.

Build up slowly.

The easiest way to start building your own emergency food supply is to purchase a couple of extra food items with your normal family grocery shop each week.

This way you won't be spending a lot of money all at once and before long, you will have your food stash ready. Aim for at least two weeks' worth of food supplies for your family to start, then, if you have room build this to one month's supply. Don't forget about your family pets. They will need to eat too!

Buy what you like to eat.

When buying and storing food supplies remember to purchase foods your family likes to eat, and you know how to prepare. Examples of food supplies that are ideal for preparing your home are included at the back of this book.

Learn to substitute.

It is a good idea to have a combination of foods in your supply. Tinned, packaged, dehydrated, fresh and frozen. Remember there is a good chance that you won't be able to *pop down to the shop* to purchase a particular ingredient so you will have to substitute.

For example, if you don't have tinned tomatoes you can make a substitute:

<u>Substitution for tinned tomatoes</u>

Mix 1 ½ Tablespoons of flour with 1/4 cup of water and whisk together until lump free.

Add another 1 ¼ cups of water, plus 4 Tablespoons of tomato paste and 1 Teaspoon of sugar.

Bring to simmer on stove until mixture thickens to your liking.

This can be used in place of 1 can of tomatoes.

Rotate your supplies.

When you first start making your emergency pantry or food stocks, make an inventory of what you have purchased and the expiration date. As you purchase more food items just add it to the list and when you use a particular food item just mark it off the list. A good way to do this is on your computer, phone, or tablet.

This is important as you can see exactly what you have in stock and what you still need to purchase. It's no good having thirty jars of pasta sauce but no pasta!

It is also a good way to see which foods may be coming up to their expiry date and need to be eaten.

Get into the practice of rotating your food supplies. Place older stocks at the front of your pantry/food storage to be used first and newer items at the back.

Keep adding newer items to the back as you purchase more.

Check the condition of your supplies.

Check the condition of your tinned/packaged foods before you purchase them. Don't buy food stuff that is close to its use by date if you arc going to storc it. You want to be able to store most of your foods for at least 1-2 years where possible.

Don't buy tins that are rusty as they can potentially allow bacteria to enter the can.

Avoid tins that are dented.

Any tins that are swollen should be thrown away.

Where to store your food

If you run out of space in your main pantry and don't have another area such as a spare cupboard to store your supplies, you can use several large plastic boxes with lids. Label the boxes with numbers and use your inventory to note what's stored inside. Include a couple of can openers!

Keep your food in a cool dry place and avoid storing food in the garage if you live in a hot, humid climate as this will degrade your food quickly.

Keep food stocks off the ground whenever possible unless stored in containers.

Be mindful of pests trying to eat your precious food stores!

Add some treats!

Don't for get to have a few treats in your food supplies.

It's not much fun having to experience an emergency/disaster especially with kids, so a few treats your family enjoys eating are a good idea. Just don't go overboard as you will probably be doing a lot of sitting around and not a lot of exercising! Loading your body with sugar will not help your immune system either.

Examples of treats include chocolate, chips, popcorn, cakes and biscuits, tinned fruit and desserts and a few bags of sweets. Yes, I know that's a lot, but you don't have to choose all of them! You can also make your own if you prefer a healthier option e.g. nut bars and granola bars.

Here is an example of food supplies for a family of four if fresh or frozen food is not available. Remember to select the specific fruits, vegetables, and meats your family likes to eat.

For three days

Vegetables: 6 cans of vegetables such as carrots, corn, green beans, peas or other vegetables.

You can also use dehydrated vegetables such as potato flakes.

Fruit: 3 large cans of fruit salad, peaches, pears or other fruits if fresh is not available.

Protein: 6 cans tinned tuna, chicken, beef, beans or legumes.

Grains: 1 package rice or quinoa

1 package pasta/spaghetti or other grain.

Dairy: 3 cartons long life milk or 1 package powdered milk.

Other:

cereal/oats

1 package pancake mix

1 box crackers/rice cakes

Vegemite/peanut butter/honey etc

Salt/pepper and herbs and spices

2 jars pasta sauce

Sugar, tea/coffee/cocoa

1 pack of granola/muesli bars

A few treats

For seven days

<u>Vegetables:</u> 15 cans of vegetables such as carrots, corn, green beans, peas or other vegetables.

<u>Fruit</u>: 7 large cans of fruit salad, peaches, pears or other fruits if fresh is not available.

<u>Protein</u>: 15 cans tinned tuna, chicken, beef, beans or legumes.

<u>Grains</u>: 2 package rice or quinoa

2 package pasta/spaghetti or other grains.

<u>Dairy</u>: 7 cartons long life milk or 2 packages powdered milk.

<u>Other</u>:

cereal/oats

1 package pancake mix

3 box crackers/rice cakes

Vegemite/peanut butter/honey etc

Salt/pepper and herbs and spices

6 jars pasta sauce

Flour

12 cans soup, stews/ready meals

Sugar, tea/coffee/cocoa

6 cans dessert

2 packs Muesli/granola bars

A few treats

For one month

Vegetables: 36 cans of vegetables such as carrots, corn, green beans, peas or other vegetables.

Fruit: 12 large cans of fruit salad, peaches, pears or other fruits if fresh is not available.

Protein: 24 cans tinned tuna, chicken, beef, beans or legumes.

Grains: 4 packages rice or quinoa

4 packages pasta/spaghetti or other grain.

<u>Dairy</u>: 30 cartons long life milk or 4 packages powdered milk.

Other:

cereal/oats

4 packages pancake mix

5 boxes crackers/rice cakes

2x Vegemite/peanut butter/honey etc

Salt/pepper and herbs and spices

10 jars pasta sauce

Flour

20 cans soup, stews/ready meals

Sugar, tea/coffee/cocoa

A few treats

Chapter Eight

What About Your Pets?

Don't forget about the needs of your furry and feathered family members! As a pet owner, it is your responsibility for the safety and welfare of your pet in the event of an emergency or natural disaster. If you plan ahead and are prepared, you can help to keep your animals safe and out of danger.

Make a pet emergency plan and pet emergency kit. Keep these with your own family emergency kit.

Remember that animals will require a constant source of food, water, shade, and a safe place to shelter during a disaster. Depending upon the emergency, for example, during a storm, pets will need reassurance (just like children!)

Keep track of how much your pet eats in a week. Slowly build up an emergency food supply for your pet by buying an extra can or pack of food each week until you have enough food for at least two weeks.

Emergency Pet Plan

An example of an emergency pet plan can be:

- Visit your vet to ensure their immunizations are up to date.

- Ensure your pets have adequate identification.

- Take a photo of your pet to assist with their identification.

- Have ready phone numbers of your veterinarian and local animal welfare agency like the RSPCA.

- Have ready the phone number and address of a friend or relative who can take your pet in case you need to evacuate. Not all emergency shelters will take animals.

Emergency Pet Kit

An example of an emergency pet kit

Enough pet food for at least three weeks. For example, dry and tinned food for cats and dogs, fish food, seed for birds, hay and pellets for rabbits, guinea pigs, mice, chickens etc.

Drinking water for three weeks.
Water and food bowls.
Pet registration or licence papers
Bedding, familiar blanket.
Pet toy and Grooming equipment.
Medications.
Litter tray and litter refills or newspaper.
Plastic bags, paper towels, gloves, and disinfectant to clean up any messes.
Leash or pet carrier in case you need to evacuate your home.

If you need to evacuate your home take your animals with you.

Birds, Rabbits Guinea Pigs, mice etc will need to be carried in cages, a secure box with lid and air holes or a pillowcase if you don't have anything else.

Fish can be carried in a large wide-necked jar with a secure lid. Fill the jar with two thirds water. When you are travelling, regularly remove the lid and use a straw to blow air into the water to aerate it.

Snakes, lizards and other reptiles will need to be carried in a container with a secure lid and air holes. If you don't have anything else, use a securely tied pillowcase or sack.

Chickens and aviary birds can be affected by smoke, so use wet hessian to cover a cage like a curtain.

Dogs and cats should be transported in pet carriers or on a leash.

If you cannot take your pets with you,

- Leave your pets indoors.

- If they must be outside do not tie them up.

- Provide adequate food and water in large heavy bowls that can't be tipped over. A slow dripping tap into a bowl can also be a source of water.

- Use food dispensers were possible to regulate the amount of food.

- Make sure all pets are properly identified.

- Provide toilet litter or newspaper where appropriate and separate bedding for each pet.

- In case of flood, position a heavy chair or crate to allow access to higher refuge such as a bench where adequate food and water should be left.

- Place your pet in a room that can be easily cleaned such as a laundry or bathroom.

Chapter Nine

What can you do for entertainment?

Okay, so going into isolation or lockdown is a great time to catch up on Netflix and other tv show/ movies you've been wanting to watch, but you can't sit and watch TV all day (well you can, but eventually you will get a headache!) and what if you don't have power? Here are some alternate entertainment ideas besides the television and computer to keep you and your family occupied.

- Playing Cards. There are numerous card games, and they can be a fun bonding experience for your family. Even younger children can play card games for example snap and go fish. And if you get sick of playing you can always try building a house of cards, that will really test your patience!

- Board games (there are some fun ones out there that cater to lovers of television series such as *Game of Thrones Monopoly and Harry Potter Cluedo*), there are also chess, checkers, and other old-style games you may have always wanted to learn.

- Yo-Yos (get the kids to take these outside or on the balcony if you don't have a backyard).

- Rubik's cube and other puzzle games.

- Jigsaws.

- Music.

- Books! Grab a few books or a series from your local bookstore.

- Magazines and puzzle books.

- Books on tape.

- A couple of new toys for the kids will keep them occupied for a few days.

- Active games such as skipping ropes and basketball that can be played with in your backyard if it's safe to go outside!

- Coloured pencils/markers and colouring books or blank books for drawing.

- Arts and crafts for the kids or yourself (maybe you've always wanted to try knitting, quilting, dressmaking or woodworking).

- Hand weights/ yoga mats/ stretching bands to do some light exercise if you feel you want to burn off some energy.

- Renovate your house – only joking! You can, however, use your time to complete all those odd jobs you have been putting off. Maybe not *entertainment* but at least it will keep you occupied!

Chapter Ten

Storms, cyclones, and hurricanes.

Cyclones, hurricanes, and typhoons can cause major damage to property and risk to life. So, what's the difference? They are basically the same thing, however, are given different names depending upon where they form. Cyclones are formed over the South Pacific and Indian Oceans. Hurricanes are tropical storms formed over the North Atlantic and Northeast Pacific Oceans and Typhoons are formed over the Northwest Pacific Ocean (www.bbc.co.uk).

These types of storms are stronger over water where the warm sea powers them, however they can also create a lot of damage over land where strong winds can flatten homes, knock over trees and power lines and tip cars. The safest place is to remain indoors as most injuries and fatalities are caused by flying debris.

What can you do to protect your family and property if a cyclone, hurricane, or typhoon is heading your way?

1. Listen to News broadcasts and emergency bulletins as to whether you need to evacuate to a safer area.

2. Have your relocation and emergency kits ready in case you must leave in a hurry. (See the appendices at the back of the book for examples of emergency and relocation kits).

3. If you are staying in your home, prepare for the forthcoming storm.

4. Be prepared for the likelihood you may lose power to your home.

5. The Government may declare a state of emergency following a storm, which means many day-to-day duties will be stopped as it focuses on dealing with the aftermath of the storm. You should be prepared for this to happen.

6. Floods and other damage can be caused by storms. Be prepared to *shelter in place* inside your home for several days to weeks. Especially if supplies/ roads etc are cut off.

Preparing your home outside

- Secure items outside your home in your yard which could act as flying debris in high winds. Items such as swing sets, bicycles, skateboards and other children's toys, barbeque grill, outdoor furniture, rubbish/trash bins, outdoor potted plants etc. Anything that is not secured to the ground.

- Keep your gutters clear of leaves to ensure they drain water properly.

- Keep any trees with dead branches pruned to avoid them falling on your roof.

- Make sure your house number is visible from the street so emergency vehicles and personnel can easily locate your house if need be.

- Know how to switch off the electricity, water and gas in case required.

- Board up your windows with plywood or storm shutters.

Preparing your home inside

Food

- If you have lost power or think you may lose power, move commonly used items such as milk, butter and eggs to an esky/cooler stocked with ice to keep them cold.

- Keep other food in your refrigerator and freezer and keep the doors shut. Some foods in your freezer will thaw quicker than others and these should be consumed first such as ice cream and frozen berries.

- Fill any empty spaces in your freezer with bags/containers of water as these will freeze and help to keep the other contents cold.

- Place a sign on the refrigerator reminding household members not to open the door. Every time the door is opened, cold air flows out and warm air rushes in raising the temperature inside.

- A full freezer will keep food frozen for 48 hours if left closed.

Cooking

Prepare your alternate cooking source (see chapter on cooking in an emergency) and extra fuel.

Lighting

Ensure you have candles, torches/flashlights etc. ready to use once the power goes out.

Emergency numbers

Have your list of neighbours, family, and emergency numbers in an easily accessible spot to use if you need to.

First Aid

Keep a first aid kit and fire extinguisher close at hand in case of any accidents. Ensure that family members know how to use the fire extinguisher and can actually lift it.

It is no good getting the biggest extinguisher you can find if no one can lift it or use it effectively. A good compromise is to have a combination of larger and smaller fire extinguishers available in your home.

Generator

A fuel-based generator can be particularly useful during a storm. If your power goes out it can be used to power a small refrigerator and light for several hours depending upon the size.

Emergency kit

Ensure you have a waterproof emergency kit for your family which includes as a minimum a battery-operated radio, torch, spare batteries, mobile phone, and charger, first aid kit, toiletries, and sanitary items. (See Appendices at rear of book for more Emergency kit ideas). Make sure the kit is easily located and everyone in the family knows where it is kept.

Cyclone warning system

Cyclones can be severe causing destructive winds, torrential rainfall, flooding and dangerous storm surges. The Bureau of Meteorology (BOM) issues cyclone information to the public in the form of cyclone watch and cyclone warnings.

Alerts are issued to advise what to do before, during and after a cyclone. The different levels reflect the increasing risk to the public.

Table 1 Cyclone Warning System

BLUE ALERT

Start preparing for a cyclone.

YELLOW ALERT

Take action and get ready to shelter from a cyclone.

RED ALERT

Take shelter immediately.

ALL CLEAR

The cyclone has passed but take care to avoid danger caused by damage.

Table 2 Other Severe Weather Warnings

Storm Surge Warning

This warning is given when there is a danger of life-threatening rising water moving inland from the sea usually within 36 hours. Listen for evacuation orders from your local officials in case you are advised to leave the area.

Hurricane Warning

A hurricane warning is usually given 36 hours before a hurricane hits the land giving you time to prepare for the storm force winds (sustained winds of 120 kmph/ 74 mph or greater). Prepare to evacuate if you are advised to do so.

Tropical Storm Warning

This warning is given where winds are expected to be 60-115 kmph/39-73 mph.

Typhoon Warning

Typhoon warnings are given 36 hours before the imminent approach of a typhoon to coastal areas.

<u>Watches</u>

Storm surge, hurricane and typhoon watches are issued when these weather conditions are expected within 48 hours.

Table 1 Hurricane Scale (www.ready.gov/beinformed/hurricanes)

Category	Winds (mph)	Damage	Storm Surge
1	74-95	**Minimal** Unanchored mobile homes, vegetation, and signs damaged.	4-5 feet
2	96-110	**Moderate** All mobile homes, roof, and small craft destroyed. Flooding.	6-8 feet
3	111-130	**Extensive** Small buildings destroyed; low lying roads cut off.	9-12 feet
4	131-155	**Extreme** Extensive roof damage, trees down, major roads cut off. Flooding.	13-18 feet
5	>155	**Catastrophic** Most buildings and vegetation destroyed, major roads cut off, homes and property flooded.	>18 feet

During a Cyclone, Hurricane or Typhoon

- Close all external and internal doors.

- Stay inside an interior part of your home away from windows and exterior doors, preferably close to a toilet/bathroom.

- Lie or crouch low on the floor under or next to a heavy piece of furniture.

- Listen to emergency broadcasts and instructions.

- Try to keep yourself and your children calm.

- Keep pets indoors with you. They will need reassurance too!

After the Storm has Passed

- Once the storm has passed and the area has been reported safe you can return to your home to survey the damage.

- It you are already sheltering in your home, ensure no one is hurt. Be alert for fallen power lines, trees and other debris close to your property.

- Check for roof damage, fallen trees and any instability in your home. If anything looks dangerous then leave straight away.

- Look for flooding or water damage.

- Take photographs and video of any damage for insurance purposes.

- If flooding has occurred, take precaution for hidden debris. See the chapter on flooding.

Chapter Eleven

Floods

Floods can be unpredictable and extremely destructive. They can isolate communities, destroy property, cut essential services, and cause injury and death.

Apart from physical damage, experiencing a flood can be an emotional time and if you are not prepared recovery can be slow. A few hours spent making your home secure, preparing a family emergency kit and flood plan can help you and your family survive the effects of a flood in your community. (See the Appendices at end of the book for examples of an emergency kit and flood plan).

Apart from flash floods, most other floods allow some warning time. In many situations, unless a major flood is expected, you may be able to keep flood water from entering your house, if you are prepared to take the necessary action. So, plan and prepare ahead of the event.

Remember, even if you take such measures to protect your home, you should still have a further action plan in case your flood-proofing fails, and you must evacuate.

Levels of flooding

The Bureau of Meteorology uses flood terms to describe levels of flooding depending upon the damage expected.

Table 3 Types of Flooding

Minor flooding: Causes inconvenience. Low-lying areas next to watercourses are flooded. Minor roads may be closed, and low-level bridges submerged.

Moderate flooding: In addition to the above, the evacuation of some houses may be required. Main traffic routes may be flooded. The area of flooding can be substantial in rural areas.

Major flooding: In addition to the above, extensive rural areas and/or urban areas are flooded. Properties and towns are likely to be isolated and major traffic routes likely to be closed. Evacuation of people from flood affected areas may be required.

Local Flooding: Used where intense rainfall could be expected to cause high runoff in limited areas local to the rainfall, but not necessarily leading to significant rises in
main streams.

Flash Flooding: Flooding occurring in less than 6 hours of rain, usually the result of intense local rain and characterised by rapid rises in water levels. Flash floods are difficult to predict accurately and give little time for preventive measures.

Preparing for a flood

- Check your emergency kit. Make sure everyone in the family knows where it is located (see Appendices at the back of this book for examples of what to include in an emergency kit).

- Prepare a flood plan of action.

- Keep a list of emergency phone numbers on display, such as your local emergency service office, police, ambulance, hospital, and essential services, for example, gas and electricity.

- Check your insurance policy covers flood damage.

- Have emergency cash available in a waterproof bag.

- Have three weeks food and water available for each family member. Don't forget your pets, they will require food and water too!

- Have sandbags ready to place at the base of exterior doors to lessen the water flowing into the house.

When floods are due:

- Monitor weather forecasts and warnings online for example at the Bureau of Meteorology (BOM). Listen to the local radio station for updates.

- Secure hazardous items.

- Roll up rugs, move furniture and valuable items to a higher level if possible.

- Place important documents, valuables and vital medicines in a waterproof container or bag.

- Raise furniture, clothing, and valuables onto beds, tables and into roof spaces were possible. Place electrical items in the highest place.

- Keep a torch, waterproof radio, and your phone with you.

- Listen for emergency warnings and instructions.

- Switch off electricity and gas supplies to your home.

- If you have a circuit breaker panel board, switch each electrical circuit breaker to the OFF position.

- Close the main gas valve. (This valve is generally located on the gas piping just prior to its entry into the gas meter).

- Gas cylinders/bottles should be tied down or disconnected and moved above anticipated flood height.

- Turn off the main water valve so flood water cannot enter the tank. (It usually is found on the main line where the water supply enters your property at the water meter).

- Place a strong plastic bag full of sand or earth in the toilet bowl to prevent a back-flow of sewage into your home. Also place a strong plastic bag full of sand or earth over shower and bath outlets.

- Position sandbags at the bottom of any doors leading to the outside of your house.

Tips for the elderly or those with special needs.

- Disabled and elderly persons will usually require special assistance as they may be dependent on the help of others to prepare their properties and evacuate if required.

- Assess your own special needs, limitations, and capabilities realistically and honestly.

- Include details of any special dietary needs.

- Write down the name, address and phone numbers of your doctor and medical specialties and give a copy to a family member, friend or neighbour who could help if required.

- Keep medications, duplicate prescriptions, and other medical needs handy.

- Keep mobility items close at hand.

- Have a mobile personal alarm with you in case you need help or assistance (these can be worn around your neck). Personal alarms send a SOS and your GPS location to the emergency services and nominated people so they can assist you.

- If you evacuate your home ensure you tell a family member, friend, or emergency worker your time of departure and intended destination.

Preparing to relocate

If you decide to relocate your family to safer, higher ground there are some things you should do first if you have time and it is safe to do so.

- Take a relocation kit with you. A relocation kit is in addition to your emergency kit and is in case your family needs to evacuate in a hurry. Items should include warm spare clothing, secure comfortable closed-toe footwear, sleeping bags and bedding, extra food and water, pet leash/ carrier and other pet requirements, personal documents, sanitary items and medications, car and house keys and any valuables that can be carried.

- Inform friends, family, neighbours, or the police that you are intending to leave your home.

- Lock the windows and doors of your home.

- Secure and empty refrigerators and freezers and leave doors open to stop them floating away.

- Turn off power, water, and gas.

- Fill your car fuel tank and stock your car with emergency supplies such as spare warm clothing and shoes, bedding, camping stove or burner, food, and water.

- Do not drive into water of unknown depth and current.

- Take your pets with you. If this is not possible place food, water and bedding on a bench, table or bed and ensure they will be able to reach it.

Travelling during a Flood

Most deaths during flooding occur when people enter flood waters either in boats, vehicles or on foot. Boating, driving, and walking in flood areas should be avoided unless absolutely necessary.

Boating in flood waters.

If you are in a metal boat, keep away from power lines and power poles. If you are in a wooden or fibreglass boat, do not touch the water or metallic parts of the motor when near wires or poles. Consider all fallen wires as dangerous.

Always wear a life jacket and carry items such as: oars, extra fuel, anchor etc.

Driving in flood areas.

Take your emergency plan and kit.

Carry plenty of food, water, and fuel.

Avoid driving in flooded areas at all costs. Enter only if essential and safe to do so and proceed slowly and steadily.

What condition is the road in? Beware of fallen power lines and floating objects.

Don't enter flood waters before checking depth and current. In just 15 cm of flowing water, floods can take control of a small car.

How strong is the current? Cars have been washed away in shallow floodwaters with strong currents.

Upon leaving flooded area, dry out brakes by applying light pressure until grip returns.

If your vehicle becomes stranded or stalls in flood water, leave it immediately and move to higher ground before the water rises further.

Avoid driving at night – potholes and clear water cannot be seen.

Let others know you are leaving.

Walking or swimming in flooded areas.

Don't swim in flood water – it is usually contaminated and often contains hidden snags, strong currents and other hazards.

If you must enter shallow water, wear shoes to protect your feet. Don't proceed beyond waist-depth unless absolutely necessary (and only if there is no obvious current).

Do not go anywhere alone.

Keep clear of fallen/submerged power lines.

Take care on foot bridges and walkways as they may be extremely slippery.

After a Flood

When returning to your home after a flood you may be surprised at the amount of damage. Essential services such as power, water, sewage, and gas services may not be working, roads may be damaged and services such as local stores, banks and ATM's may not be open.

Tips for returning home:

- Wait for the *All clear* from emergency services before going into a flood effected area.

- Be prepared for a slow journey as road conditions may have changed and some roads may be closed. Take caution.

- Before returning to your area, fill your car with fuel, stock up on food, water, sanitary supplies, and pet food. Also, any medicines or prescriptions needed.

- If your property is severely damaged, stay out until a building inspector has checked it out for safety.

- Before entering your house, wait until water has fallen below floor level.

- Use a torch to inspect any damage. Do not use a lighter, matches, naked flames or cigarettes in case of gas leaks.

- Wear rubber boots (or at least rubber-soled shoes) and rubber or leather gloves.

- Check with electricity, gas, and water authorities to determine whether supplies to your area have been interrupted and are safe to be turned on by you. Do not turn on any lights or appliances until a qualified electrician has checked the entire electrical distribution system.

- If the water supply system has been flooded, you must assume it is contaminated. If there is any chance of flood contamination of your drinking water, drink only boiled, sterilized, or bottled water until the normal water supply has been declared safe by health authorities.

- Upon entering your home look out for snakes, spiders and any other wildlife that may have taken shelter in your home. Contact wildlife rescue if need be.

- Discard all foods and medicines exposed to flood water except those in sealed (airtight) metal cans. Remove the paper labels from the cans and wash the cans in soap and warm water.

  Then immerse in a solution of three quarters cup of household laundry bleach per five litres/1 gallon of water for two minutes to disinfect the outside of cans. Rinse immediately in clean water. Do not treat aluminium cans with bleach solution. Mark the outside of the cans with permanent marker to identify the contents of the can and use by date if it has one.

- Remove and burn or bury rubbish, decaying vegetation, food, and driftwood.

- Wash surfaces that have been in contact with flood waters with disinfectant or bleach solution. This will help to reduce the danger of flood-carried infections.

- Wash your hands thoroughly with a disinfectant soap after handling contaminated articles and before eating or drinking.

- When cleaning up wear rubber gloves, goggles, water resistant clothing and enclosed footwear.

- Wear insect repellent with added Deet as flood water can attract mosquitoes which may carry diseases.

- Disinfect any cuts thoroughly and cover with a waterproof dressing.

- Seek help from welfare agencies if needed.

- If you are insured, contact your insurance agent, and request an assessment and advice before discarding, authorising repairs, or cleaning damaged or flood affected property.

- Take photographs or video of any damage to help with insurance claims.

Chapter Twelve

Tsunami

A Tsunami is a series of long waves that travel extremely fast across the ocean floor due to the sudden movement of a large body of water. They can be caused by undersea earthquakes, landslides on the sea floor or volcanic eruptions (**www.DFES**).

Tsunamis differ from regular ocean waves as they can travel at 1000 kmph/ 600 mph and unlike normal ocean waves they move water all the way to the sea floor.

Because a tsunami is a series of waves, it is important to remember that the first wave may not be the largest.

What do you do when you hear a Tsunami warning?

For a land Tsunami

- Listen for emergency broadcasts.

- Go to higher ground, at least ten metres/6 miles above sea level, or if possible, move at least one kilometre/mile away from all beaches, harbours, and coastal estuaries.

- Take only essential items that you can carry such as important papers, and medical needs.

- It may be better to walk to higher ground rather than drive if traffic is congested.

- If you cannot leave the area take shelter in the upper storey of a sturdy brick or concrete multi-storey building.

- Do not go to the coast to watch the tsunami and take photographs!

- Take your pets with you if possible.

- Inform friends/family were you will be going.

For a marine tsunami

- Listen to emergency broadcasts.

- Get out of the water and move away from the immediate water's edge or harbour, coastal estuaries, rock platforms, and beaches.

- Boats in harbours, estuaries and in shallow coastal water should return to shore - secure your boat and move to higher ground.

- Boats already at sea should stay offshore in deep water until further advised.

Chapter Thirteen

Earthquake

Earthquakes occur when the cracks in the Earth's surface called fault lines move under stress. Vibrations ripple out from where the fault lines occur and cause the ground to shake and tremble. They can also cause landslides, ground ruptures and tsunami. Flooding and fire are also possible aftereffects of an earthquake.

Earthquakes can be frightening as they can strike suddenly and without warning and cannot be controlled. Unlike other natural dangers, they do not happen at certain times of the year or because of dangerous weather.

The department of fire and emergency services (DES) suggests that once an earthquake has occurred in your area you are more at risk of another one occurring again.

By making an earthquake plan with your family you will know how to stay safe and prepared for the next big shake!

What should you do when an earthquake strikes?

Before

- Know the safe spots in your home to shelter such as under a strong table or other heavy furniture.

- Prepare your family with earthquake awareness. Drop, cover, and hold on.

- Keep an emergency kit in your home including important phone numbers and medical assistance (see Appendices at the back of the book for an example). Make sure everyone in the family knows where your emergency kit is kept.

During

- **DROP** to the ground.

- Take **COVER** under a sturdy table or other heavy furniture. If there isn't anything to get under, cover your face and head with your arms and crouch alongside a bench or near an inside wall.

- **HOLD ON** until the shaking stops.

After

- Expect aftershocks. These may not be as strong; however, they can still cause damage.

- Open any cupboards and cabinets carefully as objects may have moved and can fall on you.

- If your house has been damaged, turn off the electricity, gas, and water. Check for gas leaks. Do not light any matches or lighters.

- If the power is out, turn off appliances that were on such as heaters or ovens and stoves. These could create a fire risk when power resumes.

- Watch for any broken lights or glass.

- When exiting any building, be cautious. Check for any overhead loose bricks or other items that could fall on you.

- If anyone is injured call for emergency services.

Chapter Fourteen

Fire

One of the largest causes of death and property damage is fire. If a fire starts in your home call the emergency services. It is also important to equip your house with safety measures to help combat this disaster risk.

What are some of the things you can do to help protect your home and family against fire?

Install Smoke Alarms

Most fires within the home are from small accidents such as a frypan catching fire or a candle igniting a tablecloth. These small fires are easily managed and extinguished. However, what happens if a fire starts while the household is asleep or in another room. If you are not aware of the fire and have no warning, the fire can easily and quickly spread putting lives and property at risk.

Smoke detectors are a must have in your home.

They will provide you with early fire detection and should be installed in hallways outside sleeping areas, the kitchen, and the garage.

Smoke alarms can either be hard wired to your home electrical system or battery operated. If using the battery-operated kind, ensure you check the batteries every six months.

Have Fire Extinguishers in your home.

Another important safety device is the fire extinguisher. They come in different sizes and can be used to put out different types of fire such as electrical, oil and wood. The ABC multiclass fire extinguisher will put out nearly all fire types except chemical fires. Others will only put out combustible type fires from wood, paper etc.

Your home should have a fire extinguisher in both the kitchen, garage and all members of your family should learn how to use the extinguishers and be able to lift them. If the extinguisher is too heavy it's not going to be much use!

Remember to call for emergency services and if the fire becomes too large or cannot be put out, be prepared to leave. As difficult as it is to watch your property burn, your life should come first, property second.

Using a fire extinguisher

1. Pull the pin on the extinguisher.

2. Aim low pointing the nozzle at the base of the fire and the material that is actually burning rather than the top flames.

3. Squeeze the handle or button to release the foam.

4. Sweep from side to side aiming at the base of the fire until it is fully extinguished.

5. Try to keep your back facing a clear escape path and if the room becomes filled with smoke then leave the house immediately.

Have a Fire Blanket

A fire blanket is a compact specialised material made from fibreglass and can withstand temperatures of up to 500 degrees Celsius/ 930 Fahrenheit.
They can be used to extinguish small fires in the home or garage and to wrap around a person whose clothing or hair has caught alight.
The department of fire and safety suggests storing your fire blanket with your fire extinguisher in areas such as the kitchen. However, they should not be kept too close to a potential hazard such as above a stove.
Fire blankets should only be used once.

Be prepared to Evacuate.

- If a house fire becomes too large or out of control, or a bush fire is heading your way you will need to evacuate your home.

- While this may be a difficult thing to do as no one wants to see their property burn, your life may be at risk if you stay. Many people die from house and bush fires each year.

- When a threat such as a bush fire is approaching your neighbourhood but hasn't yet arrived, listen to the radio and television broadcasts to determine when the best time is to evacuate.

- The window of time allowing for safe evacuation may be short. You must decide whether the danger of staying is greater than that of leaving.

- Agree on a family gathering point outside the home and ensure everyone, including pets are gathered there before leaving your property. Try to keep calm and call for emergency services if possible.

- If there is time and it is safe to do so, take your folder or electronic device containing your family's personal documents with you (see the chapter on *Backing up your electronic devices*).

- If possible, identify multiple escape routes from the areas being effected by fire in case you are unable to use one or it becomes blocked by traffic or unsafe.

- Turn off gas and electricity if possible. Leave the water connected. Unplug electronics and appliances except the freezer and refrigerator.

- If you are evacuating your home, lock all doors and windows to deter looters and take your keys with you.

- Wear comfortable clothing and footwear.

- If you have time, pack your car with supplies including water, food, a first aid kit, blankets, torch, and communications devices. If you have room take your most valuable items with you. This may be money, laptop, gold coins, trophies, or photo albums. What is most valuable to you and your family is a personal choice.

- Let friends or family know you are evacuating and where you are heading. Remember to inform them if your plans change.

Bushfires and Wildfires

According to the RAC (Royal Automobile Club) Bushfires can travel at incredible speeds and a fire as far away as 20 km/12 miles can reach your home in a matter of minutes.

Have a plan of action on what you will do if a bushfire threatens your area. Making last minute decisions can be deadly. See Appendices at the back of the book for an example of a bushfire plan of action.

Bushfire Dangers

Bushfires can start suddenly and spread rapidly especially in hot windy conditions. Flames are not the only risk you face in a bushfire. There are also risks from embers, radiant heat, and smoke (Department of fire and emergency services).

Ember Attack

An Ember attack can occur before, during and after a fire front passes. It is when embers or pieces of burning bark, leaves or twigs are carried by wind and create spot fires.

Embers can land in your garden, under the gutters of your house and on wooden decks. If not extinguished your house could catch fire. During a bushfire, keep a watch out for burning embers around your home and put out spot fires immediately if safe to do so.

Radiant Heat

The hotter, drier, and windier the day is the more intense a bushfire will be and the more radiant heat it will generate. Radiant heat can cause injury, heat exhaustion, and burns. Have appropriate clothing for your family to assist in dealing with radiant heat. (See appendices at the back of book for bushfire appropriate clothing).

Smoke

Thick smoke and super-heated air can be caused by bushfires making it difficult to breath. To help with this, cover your nose and mouth with a respirator mask, wet towel, or scarf. People with asthma or other respiratory conditions should be especially careful during bushfire season.

During a bushfire emergency, services will provide you with as much information as possible. Listen to radio and television broadcasts for updated information about the situation and be ready to leave if instructed to.

There are four alert levels during a bushfire.

Bushfire Alert Levels

Advice.

Watch and Act.

Emergency Warning.

All clear.

Alerts can be found on local radio, or websites such as **www.emergency.wa.gov.au**

Advice

This warning is given when a bushfire has started but there is no immediate threat to lives or homes. Stay alert and watch for signs of a fire. Continue to monitor emergency stations for further updates in case the situation escalates. Have your emergency kit ready.

Watch and Act.

This warning is given when there is a possible threat to lives or homes. A fire is approaching, and you need to put your family's plan of action into effect. Are you going to leave or stay?

If you plan to stay, make sure you do it early while it is safe. (See appendices at end of book for an example of a *leave early plan*). Only plan to stay if you are mentally, physically, and emotionally prepared to defend your home and have the right equipment.

Emergency Warning

This warning is given when there is an imminent threat to lives or homes. An out-of-control fire is approaching extremely fast. If you haven't already prepared your home it is too late, you must leave immediately if it is safe to do so.

<u>All Clear</u>

This advice is given once the danger has passed and the fire is under control. Take care and remain vigilant in case the situation changes.

Preparing your Property

What can you do to prepare your home and property for a bushfire emergency?

Ongoing property upkeep

- Cut the grass around your property so it is 10 cm or less.

- Prune shrubs so they are not dense.

- Clean gutters of leaves and debris.

- Remove any flammable material such as wood or mulch against or near the house.

- Store petrol and gas away from the house. For example, in a shed.

- Create a minimum 2-meter gap between your house and tree branches.

On the day

- Get out your family's emergency kit (see appendices for an example of an emergency kit for bushfire).

- Turn air conditioners off but leave water running through the system if possible.

- Fill containers, basins, buckets, and bath with water.

- Soak towels and cloth in water and lay alongside the inside of external doorways.

- Take down curtains and move furniture away from windows.

- Wet down the side of your house and garden that faces the fire front.

- Turn off gas supplies.

- Regularly patrol around your home for spot fires.

- Place a ladder and torch by your home's manhole so you can regularly check the roof cavity for embers.

- If you decide to leave your property lock all doors and windows and inform friends, relatives, or neighbours that you are leaving. Also let them know when you arrive safely at your destination. (See the appendices for examples of a relocation kit and bushfire leave early plan).

Travelling during a bushfire

If there is a lot of smoke:

- Drive slowly as there may be people, vehicles, and animals on the roads.

- Turn on your car headlights, fog lights and hazard lights if you have them.

- Close your car windows and outside vents.

- If you can't see clearly pull to the side of the road and wait for the smoke to clear.

- Continue to listen to your car radio for emergency warnings and instructions.

If you become trapped in your car during a bushfire

The Department of fire and safety (DFES) gives the following advice if you become trapped in your car during a bushfire.

- Stay in your car and turn your engine off.

- Park in an area with little or no vegetation on the side of the road furthest from the fire.

- Face your vehicle towards the oncoming fire.

- Close the doors, windows and outside vents and do not get out or open windows until the fire front has passed.

- Lie on the floor and cover your body with any woollen or cotton blankets or cloths.

- Stay in the car until the fire front has passed and the temperature has dropped outside.

(Bushfire Overview - Department of Fire and Emergency Services dfes.wa.gov.au)

If it's too late to leave your property

Sheltering in your home during an approaching bushfire should be your last option. If, however, it is no longer safe to leave your home the Department of Fire and Emergency Services (DFES) suggest the following:

- Stay in the house when the fire front is passing.

- If people were expecting you to leave, let them know you are now staying.

- Take shelter inside a room with two exits furthest from the fire front.

- Make sure all doors and windows are sealed as much as possible.

- Soak towels and cloth in water and lay them along the inside of external doors.

- Keep woollen blankets handy for protection against radiant heat.

- Take down curtains and move furniture away from windows.

- Wear a respirator mask or wet bandanna/scarf over your nose and mouth.

- Lay flat on the floor to limit your exposure to smoke.

- Actively defend your property by putting out spot fires when safe to do so.

- Check the roof cavity for embers.

- Drink plenty of water so you do not become dehydrated.

- Protect yourself from radiant heat with long sleeves, pants, and strong boots/shoes.

- Remain inside your house for as long as possible. If your house catches fire and conditions become unsafe, leave through a door furthest away from the approaching fire.

Returning to your home after a fire

Bushfires/wildfires can be very destructive and similar to tornadoes can leave some houses and property untouched while devastating others.

Returning to your home and community after a fire can be very emotional and upsetting as it is difficult to know what you may find.

Do not return to your home and community until you have been given the all-clear by authorities. There may be risks of a flare up or other hazards such as gas leaks, down power lines, live electricity wires, sewage spills, fallen trees and damage to roads, pathways and bridges making the area unsafe.

If your house is damaged and you require a place to stay or financial assistance, seek help from Government Welfare agencies and support groups in your state/town.

When returning to your house be sure to wear protective clothing such as gloves and boots and be cautious of any unsteady walls and ceilings. If unsure, leave your home immediately.

If you did not have time to take your family emergency kit with you which contained your personal documents etc, when you return to your property you will need to look for important items such as

- Passport, drivers' licence, birth certificate and other identification documents.

- Credit cards, bank cards, purse/wallet

- Any legal documents or certificates

- Insurance documents

- Medications that have not been damaged by the fire.

- Personal items such as jewellery, photo albums, trophies etc

- Any personal aids such as glasses.

Removing smoke and soot from clothing

Wash soot and smoke from your affected clothing by washing in a mixture of

1 cup of household chlorine bleach

6 Tablespoons of clothes detergent

4 Litres/1 gallon of warm water

Then rinse with fresh water and let dry.

Electrical Appliances after a fire

Do not touch or use electrical appliances that have been exposed to water until they have been checked by an authorised service technician.

Food and Water

Food, drinks and medicine that has been exposed to heat, smoke or water should be thrown away. Cans and tins that are rusted, dented or swollen should also be removed. Any jars or cans that are intact can be wiped with hot soapy water, rinsed in clean water and dried.

Do not re freeze any food that has already defrosted/thawed.

(dfes.wa.gov.au)

Caring for animals after a fire

Once you are authorised to return to your home ensure any pets or livestock you were unable to bring with you are safe and not exposed to any hazards. Check they have adequate shelter, food, and water and attend to any animals. If they have suffered any injuries or trauma seek assistance immediately. Organisations such as the RSPCA, your local Veterinarian and Ranger can help you care for your animals.

If you cannot locate your animals check with your local pound, animal shelter and animal control. Take a photograph of your pet and any ownership papers if possible, to help identify them.

Your pets may find returning to your home after a disaster as distressing as you do. They may be disorientated, frightened or aggressive. When first bringing them home release them in a confined area to reduce the risk of them running away.

(Dfes -Pets and other animals)

Chapter Fifteen

Tornado

A tornado is a violent windstorm characterised by a twisting, funnel shape. They are more common in the afternoon or early evening.

Tornadoes are unpredictable and may form without any warning. They can produce winds that exceed 200-300 mph or 350-450 kph and can move in any direction. The exact location of a tornado touchdown point is difficult to determine.

Unfortunately, tornados can also develop very rapidly meaning the warning signals for an approaching tornado is only a few minutes. If you live in an area prone to tornadoes there are some things you can do around your home to help keep your family safe for when a tornado does strike.

Make a family *Tornado Plan of Action* so that everyone knows what to do during this emergency. Be sure to know where you can take cover in a matter of minutes as this may be all the warning time you are given.

At least this will give you some comfort your family has made preparation for this weather event.

If there is a **tornado watch,** it means that a tornado is possible in your area. Follow your family *tornado plan of action* and prepare in case the tornado does strike your area. It is better to have been prepared and the tornado doesn't eventuate rather than being totally unprepared and a tornado hits your home!

If a **tornado warning** is given, it means that a tornado has been spotted by radar in your area. You should take cover immediately.

Tornado signs

- Large hail with or without rain.

- Dark sky possibly greenish in colour.

- Large dark, low-lying cloud that may be rotating.

- A loud roaring sound like a freight train.
  .
- Flying debris.

- Very calm absence of wind just before the tornado strikes.
  (www.spc.noaa.gov)

During a tornado

- If you are at home take your family to the basement of the house with your emergency kit. If you do not have a basement, head to an interior room away from windows and external doors. Do not open the windows of your house as this will not avoid pressure build up and will only result in flying glass and debris.

- When the tornado hits, get under a heavy table, blankets, mattress, or anything that can protect you from flying debris. Protect your head and face with your arms. Flying debris is the most common cause of death and injury during a tornado.

- If you are in a car or mobile home/caravan get out and find a solid building to shelter in. Head to the basement if possible or a tornado shelter.

- If you are stuck outside do not try and outrun the tornado! Find a low ditch, lie face down and protect your head with your arms and hands. Stay as low as possible.

www.stormpredictioncentre.com

Chapter Sixteen

Civil Unrest and Riots

Civil unrest can be very frightening and destructive. It can occur when people become afraid, angry, or frustrated and act as a group.

During civil unrest you can expect to see lawlessness, absence of emergency personnel, rioting and increased crime. If the civil unrest is widespread there can be a breakdown in social order. Mail delivery can be halted, food stores cleared of food which then creates shortages, garbage piling up and people beginning to panic.

In an effort to control people, the Government may declare martial law and curfews may be implemented.

When civil unrest affects your community, you may need to consider evacuating to a safer location until it is resolved.

If you want to stay in your home have your emergency kit, first aid kit and medical kit prepared. You may also want to look at added security such as window shutters and deadbolts on your doors.

Continue to watch the television and listen to radio stations for any news about escalations in the unrest and which areas are affected.

Chapter Seventeen

Extreme Weather

Extreme heat and cold while not necessarily a disaster, can be dangerous especially for the elderly and children.

Hypothermia

Extreme cold weather or long periods of time exposed to cold weather especially in windy conditions or with inadequate clothing can cause a condition called **Hypothermia.** This is where the body's core temperature drops significantly. If the body's core temperature which is usually around 35 Celsius/ 95 Fahrenheit drops below 32 degrees C/ 90 F it can be life threatening.

Prolonged immersion in cold water can also cause Hypothermia as the body becomes quickly chilled. **(www.health.nsw.gov.au)**

Symptoms of Hypothermia

- Feeling cold and uncontrollable shivering. (shivering may stop as the person progresses to severe Hypothermia).

- Skin feels cold and looks pale.

- Drowsiness, slurred speech, unsteady gait.

- Confusion, tiredness, gradual loss of motor skills.

- Slowed heart rate and breathing, dilated pupils.

- As the symptoms may develop gradually, you may be unaware you are developing Hypothermia.

- Even though a person with Hypothermia's body core temperature is dropping rapidly they may begin to feel extremely hot and want to shed their clothing. This will only exacerbate the problem.

Prevention of Hypothermia

- Limit the amount of time you spend outdoors in cold weather especially if it is also windy. Wind chill can increase the likelihood of Hypothermia.

- Dress warmly in layers. Don't forget your head, hands and feet as these areas lose heat quickly.

- Stay dry. Wet clothing can chill the body rapidly.

- Get out of the cold as soon as you start feeling chilled or begin to shiver.

- Drinking alcohol can lower your body temperature further.

- Avoid over exertion when working outdoors as this can cause you to sweat which then cools your body.

- Hypothermia can also occur indoors if your home is cold. Especially for the vulnerable such as children and babies, the elderly or sick, and people with very low body fat, poor circulation, or diabetes.

Treatment of Hypothermia

- Get medical attention.

- Move the person out of the cold and remove any wet clothing.

- Warm the person especially on the chest, head, and neck areas. Use warm blankets, towels wrapped with hot water bottles or skin to skin contact. Do not massage the skin or apply heat directly using a heat lamp.

- Keep the person calm.

- Give warm fluids. Do not give alcohol.

Keeping your home warm

Loss of electricity, gas or other fuel, or breakdown of you home heating appliance during winter could cause your home to become very cold and uncomfortable to live in for any extended time. It would feel the same as if you were sleeping outdoors.

The easiest way to prepare for this is to consider what your family would need if they had to spend a night outdoors. Wool blankets, sleeping bags, duvets etc. How much you need depends upon where you live and the severity of your climate.

Having back up heating solutions in your home is also a good idea. You may only need to heat one area of your home until power/gas is restored or you can have your main heating unit fixed. Examples of back up heating include wood burning stoves, kerosene heaters and oil heaters.

When using fuel burning heaters remember to keep them away from flammable materials. This includes carpets, wood flooring, curtains, clothing, and bedding. Never leave them unattended or with children.

Other solutions to helping prevent heat from escaping from your home is to use weather stripping around doors and windows. Use double paned windows and roof insulation. Keep doors to unused rooms closed.

Cook inside. The heat from your oven can assist in warming your home. At least your kitchen will be warm and isn't that where everyone seems to congregate anyway!

Use air-activated heat packs to keep warm. These small packs are activated by shaking. They produce heat and can be placed under your clothing or in your pocket to help you keep warm. Many outdoor hikers and skiers use them in winter.

Hyperthermia

Unlike Hypothermia, Hyperthermia is an abnormally **high** core body temperature.

Heat cramps, heat stroke and heat exhaustion are all symptoms of Hyperthermia. According to the National Institute of Health, when the body is overwhelmed by heat and unable to cool itself down heat stroke can occur which can become life threatening.

Children, the elderly, pregnant women, diabetics, and those suffering from illnesses all have a higher risk of developing Hyperthermia and should be watched more closely for symptoms during hot weather.

Symptoms of Hyperthermia

- Body temperature increases significantly. For example, above 40 degrees Celsius/104 degrees Fahrenheit.

- Confusion.

- Profuse sweating or cessation of sweating in later stages.

- Hot, flushed skin.

- Faintness.

- Rapid pulse.

- Staggering.

- Dehydration and thirst.

- Headache.

- Muscle cramps

- Delirium.

Prevention of Hyperthermia

- Limit time outside in extremely hot weather.

- Wear sun protective clothing, especially a hat.

- Drink plenty of fluids during hot weather. Avoid alcohol.

- Take a cold shower or bath or place feet in a cold foot bath if feeling hot.

- Do not wear too many layers of clothing.

- Give children cold foods such as icy poles/popsicles or frozen fruit.

- Sit in front of a fan or airconditioned room if possible.

- Don't overexert yourself.

Treatment of Hyperthermia

- Move the person out of the heat and into a shady, air conditioned or cool area.

- Lay the person flat if possible, with their feet elevated or sit quietly.

- If you suspect heat stroke call for medical assistance.

- Encourage the person to shower, bathe or sponge off with cool water.

- Apply a cold wet cloth to their wrists, neck, face, and armpits.

- Give cold fluids such as water or juice. Avoid caffeine or alcohol.

- Loosen any tight clothing and remove any excess layers.

Keeping your home cool

- Close any blinds and curtains on windows facing the sun.

- Use tinted windows, awnings, and roof insulation where possible.

- Turn off anything creating unnecessary heat such as lights, televisions, dryers, and dishwashers.

- Have a back-up power source to run fans or coolers in case the electricity goes out.

- Remember to keep pets inside during extreme heat and ensure they have clean water to drink as they can suffer from the heat too!

Heat and your pets

Don't forget about your pets during a heat wave as animals can also be affected by hot weather.

What can you do to help your pets be more comfortable and keep cool during extreme heat?

1. Bring your pets inside. We have often had our dog Dusty, cat Abby and Rabbit Symmion all inside during hot days. We do keep an eye on them though and our rabbit has his own portable enclosure - no need to tempt fate!

2. If you cannot bring your pet inside, make sure they have plenty of shade and shelter and check on them regularly.

3. Provide them with plenty of clean fresh water. And remember to keep the water bowl out of the sun.

4. Never leave your pet in a closed shed, garage, or car. Like children they can overheat quickly.

5. If walking your pet be mindful of their paws on the hot pavement/ground. Walk them in the early morning or evening when the temperature is not as hot. (This will also be more comfortable for you!)

6. Do not leave your pet's food out. If they do not eat it straight away, cover the dish and place in the fridge for later. Just like human food, pet food can easily spoil in hot weather.

What can you do if your pet is showing signs of heat stress?

Signs of heat stress in your pet can be excessive drooling, panting, sweating, listlessness, and the inside of their ears becoming bright pink.

1. Move them to a cooler place.

2. Try to get them to drink water.

3. Bathe your pet or wipe them with a damp towel or sponge. Or have them stand in cool water.

4. Seek urgent attention from a veterinarian if their condition worsens or they are not drinking or improving.

Power Outages in the heat

What can you do if you have a power outage in hot weather?

<u>Be Prepared.</u>

- Keep electronic devices such as phones and laptops charged so you can still use them for a while during the outage.

- Have battery, solar or generator back up available.

- Prepare an emergency kit for your family. (see the Appendices at the back of the book for examples).

<u>What to do during the outage.</u>

- Keep any curtains and blinds closed to keep your home cool.

- Limit the number of times you open your refrigerator and freezer.

- Limit the use of your oven and stove. Cook on a BBQ outside or gas burner.

- Ensure you can move your car from your garage if it has an electrically operated door/gate.

- Check that electrical appliances such as stoves and ovens are switched off if they were in use when the power turned off. These could be a potential fire hazard if they come back on when power is restored and are left unattended. For example, when everyone is asleep.

- Take extra care when driving at night as street and traffic lights may be out.

What to do in long term outages.

- When the power is restored after a prolonged outage, be careful eating perishable food products from your fridge or freezer as the loss of cold storage may have damaged them. **If in doubt throw it out.** Food poisoning can be serious.

- Ensure your car is topped up with fuel in case fuel station bowsers/pumps are not operating in your area.

- Ensure you have sufficient cash on hand in case ATM and credit card facilities are not available.

Chapter Eighteen

Back up your electronics and documents

As most of us live our lives on our computers and mobile phones. Our precious videos and photographs of friends and family, work, and personal information, contact lists and financial information are all stored on them. Nobody wants to lose this data because of a lightning strike during an electrical storm so you should always prepare your home electronics for any power disruptions and storms.

- Always back up your important data to a thumb drive, the cloud, a portable hard drive or all three!

- Have a NID (network interface device) attached to your home to protect your home's wiring from lightning strikes by directing surges greater than 300 volts into the ground.

- Install a surge protector to protect electronics against voltage spikes and surges.

- An extra level of protection is a UPS (uninterrupted power supply) which will prevent a temporary power disruption to your computer which could cause you to lose valuable data when there is an abrupt loss of power to your computer.

- Keep an eye on the weather and if a storm is likely, unplug your computers. It is not enough to switch off at the wall, you must unplug from the power outlet or phone jack.

- Back up personal documents to a portable secure password encrypted drive (and if possible, data encrypted) that can be taken with you if needed.

- It is also wise to have a hard copy of your family's personal papers in a weather protected sleeve or envelope. In case your family must evacuate your home because of fire, flooding or other disaster, your documents will be easy to access and grab in a hurry.

Trying to locate certificates and bits of paper scattered throughout your home when a bushfire is racing towards your home would be stressful.

Table 4 Important Information to Consider Storing

Drivers licence
Passport
Birth Certificates
Marriage Certificates
Mortgage Papers/Property deeds
Vehicle papers
Insurance information
Qualifications, Degrees, Diplomas
Weapon Permits
Adoption Papers
Citizen papers
Social Security information
Addresses and phone numbers of friends, family, doctors, dentists, specialists.
Tax records
Will and deeds
Photos of family
Financial information
Pet ownership
Medical conditions
Prescriptions
Next of kin

Secure family photos

Family photos can be irreplaceable especially if you are like our family and have hard copies of old photos that were taken before digital cameras were a thing. To protect yourself from losing these valuable photographs, scan your photos onto your computer then back them up to CDs, DVDs, or memory sticks.

By scanning them you also preserve them from fading or being damaged by mildew.

Digital photos, and cell/mobile phone photos should also be backed up regularly. These should be stored in several places such as your computer, an external portable memory device and the cloud.

If you have a lot of photos or video footage use several portable external memory devices or CD's. Label each with the content and date.

If you need to leave your home quickly in an emergency such as a flood, fire, or storm, you can easily grab your saved photos and take them with you as part of your family's relocation pack.

Chapter Nineteen

Stock up on Batteries

You never know when there is going to be a power outage, so it is a good idea to have a supply of spare batteries for torches, radios, lanterns, and other devices.

Batteries should be stored at room temperature and kept in their original packaging. Putting batteries in the freezer does not extend their life. Don't leave any loose batteries jumbled in a box as it's a fire hazard to have them touching each other.

Any batteries that are leaking should be discarded. Don't mix old and new batteries and always have a range of fully charged batteries including A, AA, AAA, C and D.

There are many different types of batteries including:

Nickel-Cadmium rechargeable (NiCad). These rechargeable batteries have a long shelf life, charge quickly, and can be recharged over and over hundreds of times. The do however lose power quickly, even when not in use.

Nickel-metal hydride (NiMH). These batteries hold their power longer when not is use so are useful to have as spares. They are a good choice for devices needing a higher quality battery. They are, however, single use only.

Alkaline, disposable. These batteries are commonly sold in supermarkets and hardware stores and are easily purchased. They are single use only and not rechargeable so you will need to keep a supply of them. They are a low cost; however, they do have a risk of leaking when stored for a long time.

Alkaline, rechargeable. These types of battery are rechargeable. They aren't prone to leaking, however, they can self-discharge so even when not being used can lose their charge. They also usually need to be charged before you can use them the first time.

Lithium. These are the best performing single use batteries as they have a lower risk of leaking, have a long shelf life, and provide excellent energy. They are however higher in cost than other batteries.

Lithium-Ion Phosphate rechargeable. These rechargeable batteries have a longer lifespan and charge more quickly than other rechargeable batteries. Some models have LCD readouts for the amount of power/charge remaining. This is very handy if the day is ending and you want to know if you have enough power to get through the night. These batteries can be connected to a solar panel or blanket to recharge.

Button style batteries. These batteries are in a lot of devices; however, they are not rechargeable so you will need to keep a supply of them. Because of their small size these batteries are easily swallowed so be sure to keep them out of reach of young children.

Battery Chargers

There are a lot of different battery chargers available and you will need to choose one that matches the size battery you want to charge (many are not interchangeable).

Some *smart* chargers can read the battery and stop charging once the battery is full, others have a light that changes colour, and you will need to turn them off yourself once charging is finished.

Some battery chargers will work off your mains power, some from your car's 12-volt power outlet and some from solar power.

Battery Testers

A battery tester is a good investment if your use batteries regularly or you keep your batteries all mixed together in a box. It is a simple gadget that allows you to test your batteries to see whether they still have charge.
This can be particularly useful and takes the frustration out of taking batteries in and out of a torch trying to find ones that work!

Chapter Twenty

Assess your lighting needs.

When preparing for an emergency it is important to assess your lighting needs. In case of a power outage, you need to ensure you have adequate lighting for you and your family. This is particularly important if you have small children in the home as blackouts can be frightening.

Torches/flashlights/lanterns

Most mobile/cell phones have a built-in flashlight function; however, these are usually not very powerful and, in an emergency you will want to conserve your phone battery for phone calls and messaging.

Instead, make sure you have at least one working torch/flashlight in your home that is in easy reach if you are suddenly plunged into darkness. It is preferable to have a medium sized torch/flashlight for each member of the family including children as this will make them feel more secure.

Keep these within an easy to reach areas such as the bedrooms, kitchen, or laundry (this will depend on the layout of your home).

If you have a double story home or home with an attic or basement, place a torch in these areas too. Navigating stairs in the darkness can be dangerous.

Check your torches/flashlights regularly to ensure they work, and the batteries and bulbs are functioning. Have spare batteries available in case they need to be changed.

Have at least one powerful light as this is better for illuminating your yard, and assessing dangers such as dangling electrical wires, fallen trees, rising water and suspicious noises.

Some torches have added lens filters such as a blue filter which is good for reading maps in the darkness.

Solar Lights

Garden solar lights can be extremely useful; however, they need to be fully charged in bright light (the sun) to give off enough light to be useful. During winter or a storm, you may not be able to charge them making them ineffective. They are, however, useful during summer or in other circumstances when you are in isolation and need a power source. Remember to take them back outside during the day to recharge.

Crank lights

These lights are good for an emergency if you don't have anything else. However, they take a lot of hand cranking to power the tiny internal generator and the charge doesn't last very long so I wouldn't recommend relying on these as your only lighting source (you will quickly become tired of having to crank them every few minutes!)

LED head lights

These small lights are a good investment, practical, and very handy as they let you keep your hands free. You'll need one for each member of your household. Again, check the batteries regularly to ensure they are working properly.

Candles

Candles are inexpensive and easy to purchase from your local supermarket. They are however a safety risk and should not be left unattended or within reach of children or pets. Keep them away from curtains, long hair, and other flammable materials.

Make sure the candle holder has a wide base, so the wax does not drip onto the surface below. If using candles, be sure to have a fire extinguisher within your home in case of an accident.

Most candles do not give off a large amount of light. To help increase the light quality, place your candle in front of a mirror. The flame's reflection will increase the amount of light in the room.

Larger width candles with thicker wicks will give more light than thin candles.

Battery operated candles are also available. These operate on a sensor and light up when it becomes dark.

Oil lamps

Oil lamps are not as popular as they once were, primarily because of the odour which can give some people headaches and the safety risk.

Most hardware stores sell oil lamps, spare wicks, and globes.

To increase their light, place the oil lamp in front of a mirror.

Never leave children or pets unattended with an oil lamp and make sure you have a fire extinguisher available in your home in case of accidents.

After each use, trim the wick and clean the globe. This will maximize light output and decrease smoke and soot.

Glow sticks

Light sticks or glow sticks are a reaction called chemiluminescence. That's a mouthful!

Basically, the sticks contain hydrogen peroxide and coloured die inside a plastic tube and phenyl oxalate ester inside a glass vile inside that tube. When the glass tube is broken or shaken a chemical reaction occurs causing light.

Heat can speed up the chemical reaction so placing the light stick in a pot of boiling water will increase the light it emits. Cold will slow it down.

Unfortunately, the light from glow sticks is not very bright hence the name. They are, however, waterproof so can be used underwater. They are also a good way to keep track of family members at night, especially small children without having to use a torch/flashlight thus conserving batteries. Plus, they're fun and the kids will enjoy wearing them.

Chapter Twenty-one

Electrical Power

The loss of electrical power for a few hours can be annoying but liveable. You might miss out on watching your favourite TV show or have to resort to a cold dinner by candlelight, but when it's only for a few hours or even half a day it's bearable. The loss of power for several days or more, however, can create real hardship if you are not prepared with an alternate power source.

Power to your house is supplied by your electrical company either by overhead or underground wires in the form of AC electricity.

Other forms of AC power you can use when the power grid is down include:

Generators

A portable generator is a fuel burning engine that produces AC electricity. They usually run on either petrol/gasoline or diesel and come in different sizes.

Some things to remember when using a generator are:

- Learn how to use your generator properly and keep it maintained.

- They need to be placed outdoors when in use as like all gas-powered engines they vent poisonous fumes. A heavy-duty extension cord can be used to connect your generator to the appliance inside your house that you want powered.

- Don't operate your generator outside in the rain. Keep it dry.

- Generators use a lot of fuel so cannot be used for long term electricity needs unless you have an unlimited supply of fuel!

- Prepare a stockpile of fuel to handle your generator needs. Remember that stored petrol/gasoline will only last 6-12 months before it deteriorates. To extend this time to several years, add a stabilizer to your stored fuel.

- Never store fuel inside your house – a garage or shed is preferable.

- Store in approved tightly closed containers in a dry well-ventilated area out of sunlight.

- Before refuelling turn the generator off and let it cool down. Fuel spilt on a hot generator can catch fire.

- Don't overfill the tank. Leave space at the top to allow for the fuel to expand as it heats up.

- Don't over exceed your generator's power capabilities.

- Have a schedule of when you will use your generator during the day so as not to exhaust your fuel supply too quickly. For example, two hours in the morning and two hours in the evening.

Although this will mean your family will be without AC power for most of the day you will still be able to complete quite a few necessities for several days.

This is important as you don't know how long the power may be out for.

Some of the necessary activities you could use your generator for include cooking, heating/ boiling water, washing clothes, tuning into radio or television emergency broadcasts, charging radios, laptops, phones, and batteries, powering a light at night.

Batteries

Batteries provide DC power to portable devices such as radios, torches/flashlights, phones etc.

They can be either single use batteries or rechargeable. It is a good idea to have a supply of both kinds as each have their advantages and disadvantages.

See the previous chapter *Stock up on batteries,* for further information on the different types and their benefits.

Solar Power

Solar powered chargers are another option for an alternate energy source especially if you live somewhere with a sunny climate! They vary in size from ones you can hold in your hand to large panels and fold out blankets.

12 Volt solar panels/blankets are designed to convert sunlight into an electrical current. They can be used on their own to power appliances which are not sensitive to fluctuations in voltage such as pumps or a small fridge, or to recharge portable lithium-ion batteries. The batteries can then be used to charge cell/mobile phones, radios etc.

To power sensitive appliances such as cell/mobile phones, laptops, radios etc directly from the solar panel, you will need an inverter.

The advantage of solar power is as long as you have enough sunlight to power your solar cells, they can be used over and over not requiring any added fuel.

The disadvantage to solar chargers is that unless you have a large solar panel, they only generate a small amount of power. They also require a minimum of six hours of bright sunlight so you will need to move the solar panel around during the day to ensure it is always in the sun.

Some things to remember when using solar panels/blankets:

- Make a list of what appliances and devices you will want to power. This will help determine what size panels you will need.

- Will your back or front yard have enough sunshine during the day to charge the cells.

- If planning on using a rechargeable battery with your solar panels, ensure you get the right size. If your panels aren't powerful enough to fully charge your battery, then you're not going to get the most efficient use out of it.

- Keep your solar panel clean and free of dust to ensure the most efficient solar conversion.

- To extend the panel's life, pack it away when you are not using it.

- Will you need an additional Lithium power station or lithium-ion rechargeable battery to go with your solar panel?

- Panels using monocrystalline solar will generate more power when exposed to direct sunlight.

Lithium Power Stations/Inverter

Lithium power stations are portable devices that allow you to charge sensitive devices such as laptops, phones, and radios as well as refrigerators and lights by plugging them directly into the station. They usually have AC, USB and 240 V ports.

Power stations have built in regulators meaning you can plug a solar panel into the unit to charge it, use the cigarette lighter port in your car or use a 240 V AC port.

Many power stations have LCD screens showing you the charge level so you can see how much power you have. They also show the voltage running so you won't overload the system.

Power stations/inverters come in different size outputs. Depending upon what you want to run and for how long will determine the size you need. Obviously the larger the size the bigger the unit and greater the cost so these factors need to be considered. How much do you want to spend considering you will most likely also need a solar panel or blanket, and how much space do you have to store the unit?

Examples of appliance running times using a power station can be seen in the table below.

Table 5 Appliance Running Time in Hours

Appliance	HPS 300 W	HPS 1000 W
Laptop	5.4	21.5
Tablet	54	215
Radio	54	215
Refrigerator (medium)	2.7	10.8
Freezer	9	35
LED Light bulb	38	153
Phone Charger	27	107
65 inch LED TV	2.3	9

The best solution to provide backup electrical power for your family is to have a combination of rechargeable and single use batteries, solar blanket with inverter and a small generator. These can be purchased over a period of time. This way you are not exhausting one supply and have alternatives to choose from throughout the day and night to keep your family comfortable.

Food during a power outage

Once the power goes out you cannot be sure how long it will be out for or what caused the outage. It may only be for a few hours, or it could be for several days.

To help keep your food cold for as long as possible, avoid opening your refrigerator and freezer too often. Most food will stay frozen for 24 hours if the door stays closed.

Cook or eat the foods in your refrigerator first, especially any dairy products like milk, yogurt and cheese and any cold meats like ham and salami as these will deteriorate first.

Once any meats or seafood thaw it will need to be cooked and eaten straight away.
Do not refreeze any food that has partially defrosted.

Medication during a power outage

If you take medication that needs to be refrigerated it is a good idea to purchase a small refrigerator/cooler that can be powered by battery/generator/solar power or by plugging into your car.

Chapter Twenty-two

Communications

When a disaster strikes, your ability to communicate could mean the difference between life or death. Without communication you are not only cut off from family and friends but also from receiving information or requesting emergency assistance.

Communication can either be incoming such as television and radio or outgoing such as telephones and CB band radios.

It is a good idea to have a variety of both.

Television and Am/Fm radios

These are valuable communication tools to receive information in an emergency situation. Local stations broadcast updates and warnings keeping you and your family informed of events. Have either a battery, solar or crank style portable radio available as well as electric in case of power outages.

Scanners

Scanners are radio receivers that allow you to listen to emergency broadcasts including police, fire and rescue and the national weather service. Check that they are allowed in your country before using them.

Telephones

Land lines, mobile/cell phones and satellite phones are all useful for communication. Cell/mobile phones also allow for texting and internet searching if satellite service is available.

Purchase a phone charger to work in your car in case of power outages. Solar chargers can also be useful; however, they require a certain amount of sunlight to work.

Shortwave Radios

Shortwave radios/amateur radio operators (Ham) can act as an alternative when conventional broadcasters have gone offline. Information can be relayed by operators to communities afflicted by a disaster such as a flood.

CB Radios/walkie talkies

CB radios and walkie talkies are inexpensive short range communication devices that can be useful when phone and satellite services are not available. CB radios operate on the MHz band and walkie talkies on the UHF band.

They do not have a long range however and transmission can depend upon line of site e.g., no hills or mountains blocking the signal.

They can be a great way to keep in touch with neighbours and others in your local community.

Whistle

Yes, it may sound simple, however when you have no other means of communication a whistle may be a good way of getting another person's attention.

A loud whistle can be useful when calling for help when trapped inside a building or under rubble. Blowing a whistle takes less effort than yelling and can be heard farther away. Keep one or two in your family's emergency kit.

Chapter Twenty-three

How much water do you need?

Most of us are used to being able to simply turn on a tap/faucet whenever we want fresh water. However, sometimes a disaster or crisis can prevent this from happening. For example, when heavy rains flood water catchment areas, water can become unsafe for drinking. Local authorities may order using alternative water sources until the crises can be treated.

This book looks at what you need for a short-term crisis. Most people do not have enough space within their homes to store water for a long-term situation. A water tank or other water source would be preferable for this type of scenario.

Water consumption

If you would like to store water at your home, you need to figure out how much water you and the members of your household including pets need for a minimum of three days.

Bottled water is one of the first items to disappear from supermarket shelves when a storm, pandemic or other natural disaster is heading your way, so it is a good idea to have what you need safely stored away before this happens.

If a crisis is imminent, store as much water as possible. If you do not have containers, then fill buckets, pots or your bathtub and sink with water. Remember that water is not only used for drinking but also cooking, hygiene and sanitation.

The amount of water that is needed to support life and health depends upon several factors including age, climate, activity, and the health of the person. Priorities for water usage also varies individually and amongst cultures. For example, washing hair, or washing feet may be important to some individuals but not to others.

The quality of water acceptable for use can also vary. For example, water needed for a backyard garden or cleaning does not have to be as sanitary as water for drinking.

So, how much water does your family need? The World Health Organisation (WHO)_recommends the amount of water each person in the household requires is 7-9 litres or 1.5-2 gallons per day, which is a lot. For a family of four that amounts to 28-36 litres or 6-8 gallons per day for the household.

For a period of 3 days that figure increases to 84-108 litres or 18-24 gallons.

If family members are sick, working in hot environments or doing laborious manual work they may require more. **www.who.int**

7 litres/1.5 gallon/ 30 cups of water per day.

This includes:

2 litres/8 cups for drinking

 2 litres/ 8 cups for cooking

3 Litres/12 cups for cleaning.

If you have pets in the household, they will also need drinking water.

Conserving water

When water is scarce during an emergency or may become scarce you will want to conserve as much of your stored water and make it last as long as you can.

Recycle your *grey* water (water used for washing and cleaning) for flushing toilets, watering the garden etc. Don't use grey water on your garden if harsh chemicals have been added to the water.

If you are unable to take showers or have limited water you can take a sponge bath using a bucket of water, soap, and a sponge instead.

Antibacterial gel can also be used to clean your hands instead of water if your supplies are becoming low.

Storing tap water

Use heavy duty containers with a lid.

Do not use milk containers as these are usually made from PET (polyethylene terephthalate) which is porous, difficult to clean and only made for short-term use. Because of its porous nature, bacteria and algae can grow inside the containers when not refrigerated.

Do not use containers that have held poisons or chemicals.

Larger barrels of water can be stored; however, smaller ones are preferable. If there is a leak or the water becomes contaminated, all your water won't be lost if you have it stored in several containers.

When storing tap water in containers they need to be treated with a water preserver or used and refilled every 6 months.

Method for cleaning containers before use.

Wash your empty containers in hot soapy water, then rinse twice. Fill the container with water and 1 Teaspoon of bleach. Let sit for 10 minutes. Next, pour out the water and fill the container with clean, room temperature tap water. Store in a dark cool place. The slight residue of bleach will help prevent bacterial growth.

Purifying water

If you do not have the space to store large amounts of water or do not have access to alternate sources of clean drinking water such as a rainwater tank, another option is to purify any water sources you do have access to.

There are several methods of purifying water, some better than others. Your water may still need to be filtered if it is coming from a river or stream where rocks and sediment are present.

Chemical purification

One way of purifying water is by using chemical tablets made from chlorine or iodine. These tablets are easy to use and have long shelf lives of four years if unopened and one year if opened. When the chlorine or iodine from the tablets mix with water, they create an environment in which bacteria and viruses cannot survive. This makes the water safer to drink.

When using chlorine or iodine tablets be sure to shake your water container thoroughly to ensure the tablet has dissolved. Wait for at least 30 minutes before consuming the water.

If you find the taste and smell of the chlorine tablets unpleasant, remove the lid from the bottle or container to let the chlorine component evaporate. If using iodine use an iodine neutraliser.

Filtering the water after chemical purification can also help with the taste. You can also try adding powdered fruit drink mix that contains ascorbic acid (vitamin c).

If you do not have ready-made chemical purification tablets you can also use household bleach which is approximately 5-8 percent Chlorine to purify water. This is as effective as the chemical tablets, however not as convenient.

Household bleach also has a short shelf life of around six months to maintain its' effectiveness.

Do not use bleach that has added perfumes, dyes, or other additives.

To purify water using liquid chlorine the *Be prepared be safe* website **www.doh.wa.gov** suggests using five drops of bleach per quart or litre of water. Mix water thoroughly and let stand for at least 60 minutes before drinking.

Water that is cloudy will need to be filtered before adding the bleach.

Boiling Water

Boiling water is the optimal way of killing any microorganisms and pathogens that may be in your water. It is simple and easy to do, however, you need access to a heating source (usually gas, electricity, or wood) and it takes time to complete.

If using this method of purification, bring the water to the boil and let it *bubble* rapidly for one minute. After one-minute has passed, remove the water from the flame and let it cool naturally. You can drink the water once it has reached room temperature or is cool enough to drink. Note that the water may need to be filtered before drinking if it contains sediment or particles.

Ultraviolet light

It is also possible to purify small amounts of water using UV or ultraviolet light. An example of this is the SteriPEN, a small portable UV light pen.

Using the UV method to purify water is quick and easy. The UV light is agitated or stirred in the container of water for 30- 80 seconds disrupting the microbes' DNA and stopping them multiplying in the water making it safe to drink.

Cloudy or muddy water needs to be filtered before using a UV light as the ultraviolet will not remove dirt, particles, or chemicals.

Solar SODIS method

When no other methods of water purification are available to you, the sun can provide a good alternative. The SODIS method of purification takes advantage of the ultraviolet emissions of the sun to kill waterborne microorganisms.

Many developing countries use this method for water purification, however, to be effective you will need a minimum of 6 hours of direct sunlight.

SODIS (solar water disinfection) Method

1. First, wash your storage bottles thoroughly with soap and water including the lids and rims of the bottles.

2. Only use colourless, transparent polyethylene terephthalate (PET) bottles no larger than 2 litres in size. Glass and other plastic materials will block the sun's ultraviolet light.

3. Filter the water if cloudy, muddy or contains sediment or debris.

4. Fill the bottles with water and close the lids.

5. Lay the bottles flat and expose to direct summer sunlight for a minimum of 6 hours. Colder or cloudy conditions will require a longer time in the sunlight for it to be effective.

Filtering Water

When using water from a source such as a river, dam or stream the water should be filtered before purifying. Filtering the water will help to remove dirt, particles, and contaminants.

A filter can be as sophisticated as a shop bought water jug where water is filtered through a ceramic/carbon solid filter.

A Lifestraw filter which is a portable water filter.

Or a simple filter such as using a coffee filter paper, bandanna or muslin material or paper towels.

Making an on-the-go water filter.

Option one

You will need two water bottles.

Coffee filters, bandana, or cotton cloth.

2-3 Elastic bands.

1. Clean and air dry your water bottle or container. Once completely dry fill with water.

2. Place a coffee filter or bandanna over the opening of your second empty bottle. Secure this with two or more elastic bands.

3. Slowly pour the water from your full water bottle into the empty water bottle being careful not to damage the coffee filter paper.

4. Remove filter and purify the water with purification tablets, boiling or bleach.

Option two

You will need two water bottles with lids.

Coffee filters, bandanas, or cotton cloths.

Scissors or knife.

Sand (course)

Pebbles or gravel

Charcoal.

Small piece of foam or cotton batting

This filtering system uses a reverse osmosis type system to filter water through two bottles.

1. Carefully cut the bottom off your first bottle using scissors or a knife. You will be placing your filter material in here.

2. Cut a small drain hole in the cap of the bottle. If you do not have a lid for this bottle, cut off the top of the bottle instead of the bottom in the previous step, then pierce the bottle with several holes.

3. Place a layer of cotton batting or foam at the bottom of the bottle.

4. Break up the charcoal from a BBQ or fire into the smallest particles you can. Do not use the instant light type as it is soaked in chemicals.

5. Place the pulverised charcoal into the bottle on top of the cloth layer.

6. Add 2-3 inches or 5-7 cm of sand over the charcoal layer.

7. Then add a layer of pebbles or gravel.

8. Cover the bottom of the bottle with a piece of cloth such as a bandana, cheese cloth or coffee filter. This step is optional but will help to strain any large debris from the water.

9. Slowly pour water into the filter while holding it over the second empty bottle or container.

10. Sterilise water by boiling, using bleach, purification tablets or sunlight.

Figure 1 Home Made Water Filter

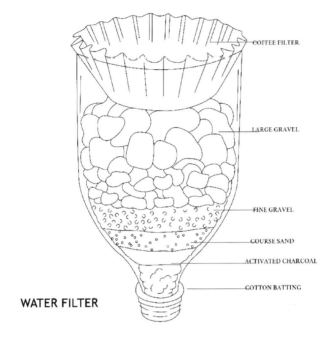

COFFEE FILTER

LARGE GRAVEL

FINE GRAVEL

COURSE SAND

ACTIVATED CHARCOAL

COTTON BATTING

WATER FILTER

Emergency water sources around your home

In worst case scenarios where you cannot access your tap water and do not have any stored water, there are alternate emergency water sources around your home you may not have thought of.

Refrigerator Icemaker

This may be a surprising place to think of looking for water, however, when you think about it a lot of refrigerators now have automatic ice makers that produce a full container of ice. You can collect the ice and when it melts you will have fresh water which is safe to drink.

Swimming Pool

Backyard swimming pools hold a lot of water that can be accessed for washing and cleaning. This water is likely to contain high levels of chemicals and organic matter so should not be used for drinking water.

Toilet

It may sound disgusting, however, the top part of your toilet – the cistern, can actually be used for drinking once purified and filtered. Scoop water out with a cup into a large bucket or container and purify with bleach or other purification means.

Rainwater

This is a great source of fresh water and can be collected in buckets, containers or even a child's blow-up swimming pool. For extra water flow place buckets beneath your house down drain spouts/pipes to collect the runoff from your roof and gutters.

While a clean source of water, the obvious problem with rainwater depending on where you live and what season you are in, is that it can be unpredictable. It may not rain when you need it or may not last long enough to collect enough water. Don't rely on rainwater as your only source of emergency drinking water.

River, Lake or Spring

Rivers, lakes, and springs are a good emergency source of water if you are near enough to access one safely from your home. Depending upon which emergency/ disaster you are experiencing, it may not be safe or advisable to leave your home.

All water from natural sources such as rivers and lakes must be purified and filtered before drinking.

Sea water and brackish water which contains a large amount of salt should never be used for drinking.

Water heater

Another source of water around the home that is often not thought of is the reservoir of your hot water heater. Many of these units are 75 gallons/ 280 litres or more in size giving you a nice emergency water supply. To access the water simply drain through the bottom of the tank.

How to drain your hot water heater

1. Make sure you turn off the electricity or gas to the hot water heater first.

2. Turn off the incoming water supply.

3. Attach a hose to the spigot at the bottom of the tank and place the other end of the hose into a bucket or large container at a lower level so it drains.

4. Open the pressure relief valve near the top of the tank or turn on one of your hot water tap/faucet in your house.

5. Open the spigot and carefully collect the water. It will be hot so take care when doing this.

6. When finished close the spigot, remove the hose, and turn on the gas/ electricity and incoming water supply.

7. Filter and purify the water before drinking.

Chapter Twenty-four

What about your car?

You never know when you are going to need your car so always keep it in good repair and get it serviced regularly. Imagine if you couldn't collect your kids from school or other activity in an impending disaster such as a severe storm, cyclone or fire? If you have prior warning of a disaster such as a hurricane heading your way, top up your car's fuel tank with fuel.

It is also a good idea to stock your car with a few emergency items in case you cannot get home, suffer a vehicle breakdown, or must evacuate from your home.

Ideas for emergency car items are:

- Car mobile phone charger.

- Flashlight/torch with spare batteries.

- Full water bottle.

- Small first aid kit.

- Folding pocketknife.

- A couple of hi-energy bars, chocolate, muesli bars or nuts.

- Woollen blanket

- Small notebook and pen.

- Small tool kit.

- Heavy duty duct tape.

- Pack wet wipes.

- Waterproof matches.

- Whistle.

Chapter Twenty-five

Cooking in a crisis

What do you do if the power goes out?
What if you have to boil water to purify it?
Do you have a back-up source for cooking? It could
be a gas stove, BBQ, wood stove, portable camping
stove or a portable Butane stove.

Fitted Gas stoves

If you have a gas stove, you will be able to use it in a
power outage. You will, however, need a match to
light the flame as the electrical ignition switch will
not work.

Portable Gas/Camping Stove

A small portable stove is particularly useful in a power outage or any situation where you cannot cook in your kitchen, for example during a flood where you need to move to higher ground. You will need either a gas bottle or butane gas cartridges to fuel the stove including a few spares. The stoves give off a good amount of heat and can be used to cook food and boil water for drinking. They are however, limited to only having one or two flames to cook on and you will need to cook in an area with good ventilation.

BBQ

A gas BBQ or grill is a handy way to cook meat, fish, and vegetables. Many of the newer variety's come with a hood making them more versatile. You can even cook a roast on them. If your BBQ is not connected to your house mains supply, you will need to keep a spare bottle of LPG gas available.

Charcoal BBQ and Fire Pits

Wood fire pits often used at outdoor gatherings can also be used to cook over. You will need an added accessory of a grill top and a good supply of wood. Food such as sausages, chicken kebabs and marshmallows can also be *roasted* over the fire pit.

Remember to take caution when using an open fire and always supervise children and pets.

Kettle style BBQs that use charcoal for smoking, grilling and even baking food are a good portable option for cooking. These should be used outside, and you will need charcoal beads or briquettes, fire starters and long matches or a fire lighter.

If you do not have fire starters you can make your own by coating cotton wool balls in petroleum jelly. Place the cotton balls at the base of the BBQ under the charcoal and light.
As with any fire be sure to take care when using and never leave your fire unattended.

Wood stoves

Wood stoves with a flat top for cooking are a useful alternative. They can be used for heating and cooking and are free until your wood supply runs out.
They do however need to be installed professionally and have a chimney or flu to take smoke from the house outside. When cooking on a wood stove you will need cast iron cookware as this will withstand the higher temperatures of the fire. You can also cook inside the woodstove wrapping vegetables like potatoes in aluminium foil to slowly roast.

Sterno Stove

A Sterno stove relies on fuel made from gelled alcohol and stored in a small can. They're portable and lightweight and can heat up tinned food quickly. You will need to have a good supply of the fuel cans on hand.

Solar Oven

A solar oven is another alternative to cooking; however, you will need ample sunlight for it to work. Foods with a high moisture content that can be cooked at a low temperature work best.

Chapter Twenty-six

How to freeze fruit and vegetables

Before freezing your vegetables, it is a good idea to cut them into smaller pieces and blanch them in boiling water for a few seconds. This kills any bacteria and slows vitamin and mineral loss.

After blanching your vegetables lay them on a sheet of baking paper to cool before placing in zip lock bags and freezing. You can then take whatever you need from the back and return the rest to the freezer.

To blanch
Fill a large pot with water and bring to the boil. Add vegetables (about two cups of chopped vegetables depending upon the size of your pot), cover, return to a boil and cook. See suggested blanching time for vegetables below.
Transfer the vegetables to a large bowl of iced water. Drain well, pat dry.

Suggested Blanching times for vegetables.

Asparagus

Prep: Trim woody ends.

Blanching Time: 2-3 minutes

To Reheat Frozen Vegetables (Microwave): 12 minutes. (Steaming): 2-3 minutes.

Capsicum/Bell Peppers

Prep: Remove seeds; cut into pieces.

Blanching Time: 2-3 minutes

To Reheat Frozen Vegetables (Microwave): 12 minutes. (Steaming): 2-3 minutes.

Broccoli & Cauliflower

Prep: Cut into florets.

Blanching Time: 3 minutes

To Reheat Frozen Vegetables (Microwave): 2-4 minutes. (Steaming): 2-4 minutes.

Brussels Sprouts

Prep: Remove outer leaves, trim stems. Halve small sprouts or quarter larger.

Blanching Time: 2-3 minutes

To Reheat Frozen Vegetables (Microwave): 24 minutes. (Steaming): 4-6 minutes.

Carrots

Prep: Peel and cut into slices or cubes.

Blanching Time: 2 minutes

To Reheat Frozen Vegetables (Microwave): 12 minutes. (Steaming): 2-3 minutes.

Corn

Prep: Husk corn and use a knife to remove kernels.

Blanching Time: 2 minutes

To Reheat Frozen Vegetables (Microwave): 1-2 minutes. (Steaming): 2-3 minutes.

Green Beans

Prep: Trim stem ends.

Blanching Time: 3 minutes

To Reheat Frozen Vegetables (Microwave): 1-2 minutes. (Steaming): 2-3 minutes.

Freezing fruit

Fruit does not need to be blanched, only washed, however stones/pits should be removed, and fruit cut into pieces.

<u>Blackberries, Blueberries & Raspberries Prep:</u>
Wash and pat dry.
Blanching Time: N/A

<u>Nectarines, Peaches & Plums</u>

Prep: Remove pit; cut into sixths.
Blanching Time: N/A

<u>Strawberries</u>

Prep: Remove the stem and hull. Cut large ones in half.
Blanching Time: N/A

<u>Lemons</u>

Prep: Remove skin and quarter.
Blanching Time: N/A

<u>Limes</u>

Prep: Remove skins and quarter.

Chapter Twenty-seven

What about MRE's?

What are MRE's?
MRE's is the abbreviation for *Meals, Ready-To-Eat*. They were initially used in the armed forces as provisions and are also widely used as a food source for emergency relief.

These *meals in a bag*, are relatively light to carry, contain about 1200 calories, are temperature resistant and are convenient. They don't need refrigeration and can be eaten straight from the packet.

Because of their long shelf life (usually 3-5 years), variety and ease of storage, many preppers now include at least a few MRE's in their food stores.

Keep your MRE's unopened in a waterproof container and remember to rotate them just like any other food item.

If you have MRE's that are about to expire, take them on your next camping trip or have fun trying them out with the kids to see which ones you prefer.

MRE's can be purchased from army surplus stores and some camping stores. Check the use by date before you purchase as you want to be able to store them for at least a couple of years until the expiry date.

Chapter Twenty-eight

Freeze Dried and Dehydrated Food

Freeze dried and dehydrated food are a great addition to your long-term food storage supplies. They have an exceptionally long shelf life, and you can make your own dehydrated food at home.

Freeze dried food.

Similar to MRE's are freeze dried foods.

Freeze dried food means the food has gone through a flash freezing process, then heated until the ice evaporates removing all moisture from the product.

These lightweight pre-prepared meals also have a long shelf life of 7-10 years and are quickly rehydrated by adding hot water to the bag or tin they are packaged in.

Freeze dried foods come in a large variety and entire meals are often freeze dried in a single package such as spaghetti Bolognese, chicken curry, beef stroganoff and apple crumble. The meals are already precooked before they were frozen so take little time to prepare. They also lose very little of their flavour and nutrients.

Store your freeze-dried foods in waterproof containers and rotate when necessary. Many camping and outdoor stores sell freeze dried foods making them easily available to the public.

Dehydrated food

Dehydrated food means the water has been completely dried out of the food without cooking it completely. This may sound uninviting; however, it means that the food stays fresher for longer.

Dehydrated food takes up less space than canned foods and is less expensive than freeze-dried food, however, it needs liquid to rehydrate and make it edible.

You can dehydrate your own fruit and vegetables at home by using the sun or a food dehydrator. Once dehydrated, store your food in airtight containers with an oxygen sachet or vacuum seal in plastic.

How to use and cook dehydrated food

Many dehydrated foods such as apples, bananas, blueberries, and pineapple can be eaten straight from the packet as a snack or added to cereal. Some dehydrated vegetables such as green beans can also be eaten *as is*, just add a little salt for flavour if required.

To cook with dehydrated food you will first need to rehydrate it and season.

Boil water (approx. 1 cup for each ½ cup of food) in a pot and add the dehydrated food. Cook until just tender. Add salt and pepper, chilli, or other spice to flavour.

Some dehydrated foods such as vegetables will only take a short time to cook. Others such as beans may take longer.

Chapter Twenty-nine

Storing Food

How to store food

If you have room in your home, you can store some of your foods in bulk. I recommend storing foods your family likes to eat a lot of such as rice, pasta, flour, beans etc. It is not beneficial to store a ton of peas because you bought them on sale if your family hates eating peas. If you hate eating peas in everyday life, you will hate eating them even more if you have to eat them every day during an emergency!

Mylar Bags

One way to store food is in Mylar bags. When used in conjunction with oxygen absorbers and food grade storage buckets Mylar bags are very efficient at creating a barrier to heat, light, moisture, and oxygen.

Thickness

When using Mylar bags use the thickest you can find. They are measured in mls. The thinner the bag the more likely food may poke through such as pasta or spaghetti.

Flat bottoms

Buy bags with flat bottoms and an added zip lock top. The flat bottom means they can stand upright which is a great help when filling your bag.

If the bags do not have a flat bottom, they will have to be propped up against something. Filling a bag only to have it fall over and spill its contents all over the floor is not much fun!

What do you need?

Mylar Bags

Food grade buckets with sealable lids

Oxygen absorbers 300-550 grams

Iron or hair straightener/tongs

Flat surface for ironing and piece of carboard

Permanent markers for labelling

Labels or masking tape to label buckets

Measuring cup or scoop

Bay leaves

I recommend using 3 kg/ 1 gallon Mylar bags to store your food. You can use larger bags, however, remember they are harder to carry and once opened the contents need to be used. Also, if all your food is in one or two larger bags and they become spoiled you will have lost a lot of food all at once.

Method

Before you start make sure you have everything ready and enough food to fill your mylar bags. You need to work fairly quickly because as soon as you open your bag of oxygen absorbers they will begin working.

- Place your iron on the hottest temperature.

- Label each of your Mylar bags with the food you will be storing and the date. Then, open all your bags and get them ready to fill. Have all your food ready as well.

- Place one oxygen absorber in the bottom of each Mylar bag.

- Add the food you are storing (about 12 cups) into each bag.

- Then add another oxygen absorber on top of the food and one Bay leaf. There should be about 2.5 cm/1 inch clearance from the food to the top of the bag.

- Lay the bag flat and line up the tops of the bag. Iron across the top leaving a small opening in one corner (this is easier done with two people. One to hold the bag and the other to iron). Do not try and fold the top of the bag as it will not seal well. Hair straightening tongs can also be used to seal the bag as they heat to high temperatures. Be careful not to burn yourself when using these or an iron.

- *Burp* the bag to let out any air through the corner gap. Then, iron across the gap to seal.

- Place your filled and sealed bag into your food grade container. Add other packaged and labelled Mylar bags until the container is full. Seal bucket and label, with the contents, number of bags and date packed.

- If you are using large bags you can place them inside your food buckets before filling so you don't have to lift them.

- Unused oxygen absorbers can be placed in an airtight jar for later use. This needs to be done straight away as they will start to absorb oxygen as soon as you open the packet.

Do not use oxygen absorbers to store sugar as they can make the sugar form a rock-hard block!

Remember, Mylar bags are not rodent proof so to stop mice and rats nibbling at your bags, place the sealed bags inside plastic containers with sealable lids.

As with your other food stores you will need to check expiry dates and use when necessary.

(https://www.alloutdoor.com)

Figure 2 Sealing a Mylar Bag with a Hot Iron

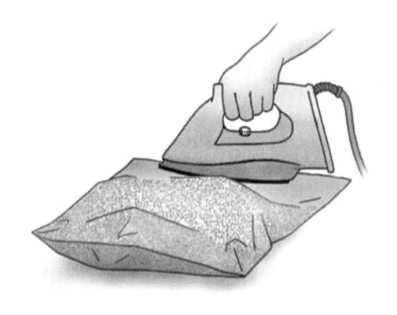

Reusing Mylar Bags

High quality Mylar bags can be reused a few times over. I simply cut the top off the bag, remove the contents, then, wash the bag and allow to completely dry. You can then reuse the bag again by filling, adding new oxygen absorbers and ironing the top shut.

Every time you reuse the bag, it will get a little bit smaller because you need to cut off the sealed portion. However, if you can reuse the bag 3 or 4 times.

What can you store in Mylar bags?

The best foods to store in Mylar bags if you are interested in long term storage (over five years) is dry and low-fat foods.

Dehydrated fruit and vegetables

White flour

Grains and white rice

Pasta and noodles

Dried Lentils and split peas

Dried beans such as red kidney, chickpea, lima and pinto

Instant coffee

Tea

Spices and herbs

Cereals such as rolled oats, corn, and wheat flakes.

Potato flakes

Foods that don't store very well for long periods are nuts and seeds, brown rice, wholemeal flour, brown sugar, dried meats and fresh foods. You can still store these in your Mylar bags with oxygen absorbers but only for 1-2 years depending upon the food.

Enemies of food storage

Light

Light can degrade the taste and quality of your food. Keep food stored in a dark area out of sunlight.

Heat

Heat can also affect the preservation of food lowering its shelf life. Food should be stored below 22 degrees C/ 72 degrees F where possible.

Do not store your canned food next to any heat sources.

Humidity

Humidity can negatively affect the taste, texture, and quality of food. Use oxygen absorbers where possible.

If you live in a humid climate, keep food stored in shelves above the ground.

Oxygen

Oxygen can increase the spoilage of food. Use oxygen absorbers where possible and seal lids tightly to keep as airtight as possible.

Pests

Mice, rats, weevils', and cockroaches can all get into your precious food and cause havoc. Keep food stuff off the floor where possible. Keep your storage area clean and use bay leaves and rosemary sprigs in your storage area to deter pests.

Inaccessibility

Make sure you can actually reach your food supplies! If food is stacked away in an area of your house that is difficult to get to you will be less likely to check your stock and rotate your food supplies. This increases the likelihood of food becoming out of date and unusable which defeats the whole purpose of having an emergency food supply! You want to be able to access your food when you need it.

Freezing Food

Another way to store food is in a large chest freezer.

You can freeze all kinds of food, however, not all food freezes well. See the chapter on *Freezing fruit and vegetables* to see which ones I recommend for freezing. For example, lettuce becomes a limp mess when frozen then defrosted (trust me I've tried it and it's not good!)

As with your other food supplies you will need to rotate your food and eat the oldest produce first. Don't just keep adding fresh food on top of what is already there, or you will quickly end up with food that is close to its use by date frozen and forgotten at the bottom of your freezer. If you are feeling really organised, you can make a running list of what you have in your chest freezer and the use by dates. I must admit I haven't done this, but it is something I would like to get around to doing.

Freezing your own prepared meals

One way to save money is to prepare your own meals and then freeze them. Good examples are chilli, spaghetti Bolognese sauce, vegetable curry and beef stew.

Use Ziplock bags to freeze the meal in portions and lay flat in your freezer. This way you can easily store more and only take out what you need. Remember to label the bags with the contents and the date the meal was made.

Tips on freezing

When using frozen foods such as cooked meals, meat, and seafood, defrost them in the refrigerator or microwave before using. Frozen fruits and vegetables can be used in cooking or in smoothies and soups.

Never re freeze partially defrosted food. Once the food has started to thaw is must be cooked and consumed.

All foods have different lengths of time they can be safely frozen. For example, bread can only be frozen for about one month whereas raw egg whites can be frozen for up to 12 months! See the table below for recommended freezing periods for different types of food.

Table 6 Safe Storage Times for Frozen Food

Product	Freezer Time
Raw Meats	3-6 months
Cooked Meat	1-2 months
Raw Chicken	3-6 months
Cooked chicken	3-4 months
Raw Shellfish	3-6 months
Cooked Shellfish	3 months
Raw Fish	2-3 months
Cooked Fish	1-2 months
Ready Prepared Meals	3-4 months
Home Cooked Meals	2-3 months

Product	Freezer Time
Soup	2-3 months
Bread/pastries	1 month
Hard Cheese grated	3-4 months.
Fruit and Vegetables	6-12 months
Ice cream	2 months
Raw Egg whites	12 months

Storage Space

One question you will need to ask yourself early on in your planning is where you are going to store your supplies.

Pantry

If you have a large pantry in your home, you may be able to rearrange your food or add extra shelving so you have an area dedicated to storage/prepping.

Basement

Basements are usually cool and dark which makes ideal conditions for food storage; however, you have to be careful of pests and damp when using your basement for storing food. Raise your food stocks above the ground on shelving to help prevent mould.

Garages, Sheds and Attics.

Garages, sheds and attic spaces are usually not the best places to store your food supplies as they can have varying temperatures and may have pests such as mice. They can be used to store other supplies such as camping stoves, torches, and candles.

Small Spaces

Other small spaces in your home you may not have considered for storing your supplies are under your bed in plastic containers on rollers, beneath the stairs, or in your wardrobe/closets.

Chapter Thirty

Face masks, respirators, and air purifiers

Air supply can be affected by numerous disasters including a volcanic eruption, industrial accident, biological agents, bushfires, and an airborne pandemic.

Protecting your family from these disasters requires insulating them from the contaminated air as much as possible. Masks, respirators, air purifiers and a well-sealed shelter all help in this regard.

Face masks and respirators have been shown to be effective at preventing the spread of respiratory illness and assisting with breathing during situations such as a large bushfire or volcanic eruption. But what is the difference between them?

Face Masks

Face masks such as the ones used in food preparation and medical facilities typically consist of a cloth material that covers the nose and mouth and ties around the back of the head or over the ears. They may be straight or in a pre-moulded form or have a wire above the nose to fit more securely.

While they protect the wearer from blood and bodily fluids, they do not protect the person adequately from small airborne particles or gases.

Respirators

Respirators are a more efficient protective *mask* usually certified by the National Institute of Occupational Health and Safety. They are designed to protect from chemical, biological, and small airborne particles.

People with beards or thick moustaches may find it difficult to use respirators as facial hair prevents adequate sealing.

Respirators can be single use or reusable models with replaceable filtering cartridges. They may cover the whole face or only the nose and mouth.

Particulate Filtering Respirators

Examples of particulate filtering respirators are the N 95 and N 99. They remove 95 and 99 percent of airborne particles.

Particulate filtering respirators commonly use material such as plastic, glass or wool to capture contaminates from the air as they pass through the filter. It is important to note that these filters cannot be cleaned adequately and should be disposed of after each exposure and replaced with a new filter.

These respirators will protect against airborne particles such as during a pandemic, fire, or volcanic eruption, however, they will not protect against gases or vapours such as a gas leak or chemical spill.

When taking into account cost and wearability, this type of respirator (for example, the N 95) will usually provide sufficient protection from airborne contaminants for most families.

Gas Masks or Air Purifying Respirators

These types of respirators usually cover the entire face and provide a much higher level of protection against chemical, biological, and nuclear contamination.

They are what is called a negative pressure device which means they require the wearer to force air through the filtration system by breathing in and out.

Due to the higher costs and wearability children may find them frightening and uncomfortable to wear. Air Purifying Respirators may not be practical for most families.

Air Purifiers

A portable high efficiency particulate air purifier (HEPA) is a good way to help purify the air in your safe room. They have been shown to remove a significant number of small airborne contaminants (99.97 percent) and are routinely used in hospitals and health centres to remove bacteria and viruses from the air. (Centre for Disease Control and Prevention).

Portable HEPA air purifies are rated according to the amount of clean air it can provide or the *clean air delivery rate* CADR. The higher the CADR the more frequently the air is cycled through the room.

Sheltering in place

To create a mini shelter in your home or *sheltering in place* you will need thick plastic sheets and thick duct tape.

What do you do?

- Select a room that can be sealed off to serve as your family's shelter. A room with an adjacent bathroom is a good idea.

- Stock your room with food, water, blankets, first aid kit, radio, television, telephone, medications, something for entertainment like a pack of cards or jigsaw. You will also need food and toiletry requirements for your pet.

- Turn off air conditioning or heating that uses circulation systems in your home. Close and lock all exterior doors and windows.

- Cover all the doors, windows, and air vents in the safe room with plastic sheeting and secure with heavy duct tape. Ensure you cut the sheeting larger than the doors and windows so that you have enough to tape down.

- When directed by emergency services gather your family and pets in your room. If you do not wish to have your pets in the room with you, just bring them into the house.

- Use a portable HEPA air filter to help purify the air in the safe room.

- Put on protective masks or respirators if required.

- Listen to the radio/ television for updates on the situation and further instruction. Officials may call for an evacuation of the area if the disaster/situation escalates so be prepared to evacuate if necessary.

Chapter Thirty-one

First aid

Medicines

Like your food supplies you should have a stock of your essential medicines that will last at least three weeks. Remember to check the expiry dates periodically and rotate when possible – newest to the back, oldest to the front.

Prepare for medical emergencies.

To better prepare your family for medical emergencies you should consider the following:

- Ensure all adults and older children in the family learn basic first aid.

- Teach everyone in the family including children how to call for emergency medical assistance.

- Each country has their own medical emergency number. Know your own country's number. It may not be the one you often see in the movies!

- Have well stocked, easily accessible first aid kits in your home and in your car.

- Know the route to your nearest emergency medical facility.

Examples of emergency phone numbers

Australia 000
Canada 911
China 120
Europe and many parts of Asia 112
Japan 119
New Zealand 111
UK 112 or 999
USA 911

When to call for help

There are many health conditions that require emergency medical services. Whether you are suffering from a condition yourself or have witnessed another person suffering a condition, always call for emergency assistance if you feel you need help.

Some examples of when to call for emergency services include:

- Unconsciousness
- Chest pain
- Difficultly speaking
- Bleeding that will not stop
- Severe abdominal pain
- Sudden changes in vision
- Sudden weakness or numbness in the face, arm, or leg
- Severe shortness of breath
- A major injury such as broken limb of head trauma
- Unexplained confusion or disorientation
- Coughing or vomiting blood
- Bloody diarrhea
- Severe reaction to an insect bite, medication, or food
- Heat stroke
- Hypothermia that cannot be alleviated

- Severe headache or migraine that will not dissipate.

Not all situations and conditions will require emergency medical assistance and many minor accidents or illnesses can be treated in the home. However, there may also be times when you will need to handle medical emergencies on your own until trained help arrives.

Before you can treat someone, you should be aware of the **five first aid priorities:**

1. Assess the situation. Don't put yourself or the patient in any additional danger.

2. Prevent cross contamination by ensuring you have clean hands, equipment and wear protective clothing if needed for example, gloves and mask.

3. Reassure the patient and keep them calm.

4. Administer lifesaving treatment first before taking other actions. E.g., stop bleeding, clear airways, administer CPR.

5. Call for emergency medical assistance if you feel you need to even if the patient is reluctant for you to do so.

Chapter Thirty-two

Minor conditions and treatments

Burns

Burns are classified as either first, second or third degree depending upon the severity or depth of the burn with third degree being the worst.

First degree burns.

This type of burn is superficial, damaging only the outermost layer of skin. An example is sunburn.

Symptoms
Red skin
Swelling
Painful.

Treatment

1. Immediately cool the burn by holding the area under cool running water for ten minutes. If this is not possible, soak the affected area in cool water or apply a cold compress. Do not apply ice directly to the skin or use any ointments or creams.

2. Give paracetamol or over the counter pain relief if required.

3. Watch for signs of infection, fever, or oozing. If infection is suspected seek medical attention.

4. If the burn covers a large portion of skin seek medical attention.

Second degree burns.

Second degree burns are a partial thickness burn where damage is down to the second layer of skin called the dermis.

Symptoms
Blisters
Intensely red skin which can also be blotchy.
Pain
Swelling

Treatment

If the burn is smaller than 8 cm/ 3 inches treatment is the same as a minor/ first degree burn.

If the burn area is larger than 8 cm/3 inches or located on several areas treat as a major burn and seek medical attention.

Third degree burns.

Third degree burns are a major thickness burn where damage is to all layers of skin and even down to muscle and bone.

Symptoms
Area may appear pale, waxy, or charred.
Pain

Treatment

1. Third degree burns require immediate medical attention. Call emergency medical phone number.

2. Cool area by flooding the entire area with cool water.

3. Do not touch the injured area. Remove any watches or jewellery that might become constrictive if swelling occurs.

4. Do not attempt to remove clothing. Wait for medical advice.

5. Reassure patient and treat for shock if necessary.

6. If patient stops breathing administer CPR.

Cardiopulmonary Resuscitation CPR

Cardiopulmonary Resuscitation or CPR as it is more commonly known is a lifesaving treatment for someone who has stopped breathing and/or have stopped breathing.

If you need to perform CPR try to remain calm, you could be helping to save a person's life.

CPR involves chest compressions and mouth-to-mouth (rescue breaths) that help circulate blood and oxygen in the body. This can help keep the brain and vital organs alive.

You should start CPR if a person:

- is unconscious.

- is not responding to you.

- is not breathing or is breathing abnormally.
St John's Ambulance (stjohn.org.au.)

Recommended Actions

DRSABC

> **Danger**. Make sure there is no danger to yourself or the patient. For example, live electrical wires.

Response. Check for a response. Ask if they are ok? And squeeze their shoulder. (You want to make sure they are not just sleeping!).

Send. If the person does not respond, ask someone to send/call for emergency assistance while you commence CPR. Do not leave the patient.

Airway. Check their mouth and throat is clear. Remove any obvious blockages in the mouth or nose, such as vomit, blood, food, or loose teeth, then gently tilt their head back and lift their chin. Check the person is breathing by using the *look, listen, feel method*. Look for chest motion, listen for breathing, feel for breath on your cheek.

Breathing. Check to see if the person is breathing abnormally or not at all. If the person is breathing, then place them on their side in the recovery position. If not breathing, then commence CPR.

1. Place the patient on their back and kneel beside them.

2. Place the heel of your hand on the lower half of the breastbone in the centre of the person's chest. Place your other hand on top of the first hand and interlock your fingers.

3. Position yourself above the patient's chest. Using your body weight (not just your arms) and keeping your arms straight, press straight down on their chest by one third of the chest depth about five cm/two inches.

4. Release the pressure (Pressing down and releasing is 1 compression).

Mouth to Mouth/ Rescue Breathing

1. Open the person's airway by placing one hand on the forehead or top of the head and your other hand under the chin to tilt the head back.

2. Pinch the soft part of their nose closed with your index finger and thumb.

3. Open the person's mouth with your thumb and fingers.

4. Take a breath and place your lips over the patient's mouth, ensuring a good seal.

5. Blow steadily into their mouth for about 1 second, watching for the chest to rise.

Following the breath, look at the patient's chest and watch for the chest to fall. Listen and feel for signs that air is being expelled. Maintain the head tilt and chin lift position.

6. If their chest does not rise, check the mouth again and remove any obstructions. Make sure the head is tilted and chin lifted to open the airway. Check that yours and the patient's mouth are sealed together, and their nose is closed so that air cannot easily escape.

7. Take another breath and repeat.

Give 30 compressions followed by 2 breaths.

If you can't give breaths, doing compressions only without stopping may still save a life. If only doing compressions, perform 100 compressions per minute.

Keep going with 30 compressions then 2 breaths until:

- the person recovers. Stay with them until medical personnel arrive.

  or

- it is impossible for you to continue because you are exhausted.

  or

- the ambulance arrives.

To carry out chest compressions on a baby:

1. Lie the baby/infant on their back.

2. Place 2 fingers on the lower half of the breastbone in the middle of the chest and press down by one-third of the depth of the chest (you may need to use one hand to do CPR depending on the size of the infant).

3. Release the pressure (pressing down and releasing is 1 compression).

Mouth to Mouth/ Rescue Breathing on a Baby

1. Tilt the baby/infant's head back very slightly.

2. Lift the baby/infant's chin up, be careful not to rest your hands on their throat because this will stop the air getting to their lungs from the mouth-to-mouth.

3. Take a breath and cover the baby/infant's mouth and nose with your mouth, ensuring a good seal.

4. Blow steadily for about 1 second, watching for the chest to rise.

5. Following the breath, look at the baby/infant's chest and watch for the chest to fall. Listen and feel for signs that air is being expelled.

6. If their chest does not rise, check their mouth and nose again and remove any obstructions. Make sure their head is slightly tilted to open the airway and that there is a tight seal around the mouth and nose with no air escaping. Take another breath and repeat.

Electrical Shock

Major electrical shock can cause cardiac arrest, respiratory failure, burns, loss of consciousness.
If you see someone being shocked or you suspect has been shocked use extreme caution when approaching them to prevent injury to yourself. Electricity can arc from person to person or from object to person if you get too close.

Recommended Action for Electric Shock

1. Carefully assess the situation for danger. Do not touch the person until you are sure they are no longer being shocked. Turn off any electrical equipment and unplug if it is safe to do so. Throw the circuit breaker. If that is not possible use a non-conducting object such as a wooden broomstick to push the source away from the person.

2. Check to see if the person is breathing. If they are not breathing administer CPR and call for emergency medical assistance.

3. If the person is breathing but injured, treat for shock by laying them down and elevating their feet. Call for emergency medical assistance.

Fainting

Fainting causes a brief loss of consciousness caused by a temporary reduction in blood flow to the brain.

Dehydration, exhaustion, lack of food, emotional stress, pain, heat and standing or sitting for long periods in the same position can all cause fainting.

Recommended Actions for Fainting

1. If someone feels faint, ask them to sit or lay down with feet elevated if possible.

2. If a person faints, check they are breathing.
   a. If they are not breathing, administer CPR and call for emergency medical assistance.
   b. If they are breathing, lay person on their back and elevate their feet to assist blood flow back to the brain. Loosen any tight clothing.

3. Once they regain consciousness, have them rest a moment before slowly standing.

4. If they do not regain consciousness, call for emergency medical assistance.

Fever

The average person's body temperature is about 36 degrees C or 98.6 degrees F. This can vary slightly between people especially if children, elderly or pregnant.

A person with a temperature above degrees 38 degrees C or 100 degrees F are considered to have a fever.
Fevers are usually cause by a virus or bacterial infection.

Recommended Actions for a Fever

1. Keep the person cool and comfortable.

2. Give the person cool water or juice to drink. No alcohol or caffeine.

3. Treat with fever reducers or pain medication such as ibuprofen, or aspirin as needed.

4. Seek medical assistance if a baby has a fever, a child younger than two has a fever longer than one day, or a child older than two has a fever longer than three days.

5. If an adult has a fever longer than three days or a temperature of more than 39.5 degrees C or 103 degrees F seek medical assistance.

Fracture/Broken Bones

Fractures or broken bones can be *compound* where they break the surface of the skin or *simple* where the skin remains intact. All fractures will require medical attention.

Symptoms of a fracture

- Bleeding.

- Swelling.

- Bruising.

- Pain.

- Deformity.

- Difficulty moving the limb.

Recommended Actions for Fractures

- If the fracture is on the arm, hand or foot and there is no bleeding, immobilize the limb using a sling or splint. Apply a cold pack to the area and seek emergency medical attention.

- If the fracture is elsewhere on the body immobilize as best as possible, have the patient keep still and seek emergency medical attention.

- If there is bleeding, carefully apply pressure to the wound with a clean cloth or bandage. Keep area immobilized and seek emergency medical attention. Do not try and push the bone back into place yourself.

- If the patient feels faint, treat them for shock by laying on their back with feet elevated.

Gastroenteritis/Stomach Flu

Gastroenteritis or stomach flu can be caused by viruses, food or water borne bacteria and stress. Symptoms may only be for 24 hours or may last longer depending upon the cause.

Symptoms of Gastroenteritis

- Nausea
- Vomiting
- Diarrhea
- Fever
- Abdominal cramps

Recommended Actions for Gastroenteritis

Give the patient plenty of liquids to prevent dehydration. Water or drinks with electrolytes are best.

Once the person begins to feel better, eat only plain foods such as crackers, boiled rice, toast, chicken soup. Avoid dairy foods, alcohol, caffeine, and fatty foods.

Children may like to have an icy pole/iced lolly.

Do not give anti-diarrheal medication unless absolutely necessary such as during travel as this can prolong the condition.

Seek medical attention if there is:

- Blood in the stool.
- High fever develops.
- Vomiting persists for more than two days or turns bloody.
- Diarrhea that persists for more than a week.
- Child shows signs of dehydration.

Head Trauma

Minor head scrapes and cuts can be treated by cleaning the wound, applying antiseptic spray or cream, and wrapping the head with a bandage.

If bleeding, apply a gentle pressure for twenty minutes.

If head trauma is more serve or bleeding won't stop seek emergency medical attention.

If any of these symptoms occur within twenty-four hours of the head trauma or at the time of the trauma seek emergency medical attention:

- Severe bleeding
- Bleeding from nose or ears
- Severe headache
- Confusion
- Loss of consciousness or breathing.
- Loss of balance
- Vomiting
- Unequal pupil size
- Slurred speech
- Seizure/fit

While waiting for emergency personal keep the person comfortable and calm. Stop any bleeding if possible, by applying a clean cloth or bandage to the wound and applying gentle pressure.

Apply CPR if person stops breathing.

Heat Exhaustion

Heat exhaustion can be caused by over heating or over exertion in hot conditions.

Symptoms of Heat Exhaustion

- Dizziness
- Nausea
- Rapid heartbeat
- Heavy perspiration
- Anxiety
- Headache
- Dark urine
- Muscle cramps
- Dehydration
- Fatigue
- Poor coordination

Recommended Actions for heat exhaustion

- Move the person out of the heat and into a shady, air conditioned or cool area.

- Lay or sit quietly. Lay the person flat if possible, with their feet elevated.

- If you suspect heat stroke call for medical assistance.

- Encourage the person to shower, bathe or sponge off with cool water.

- Apply a cold wet cloth to their wrists, neck, face, and armpits.

- Give cold fluids such as water or juice. Avoid caffeine or alcohol.

- Loosen any tight clothing and remove any excess layers.

Heat Stroke

Heat stroke is a progression of heat exhaustion and can be dangerous if not treated.

Symptoms of heat stroke

- Elevated body temperature of 40 C/ 104 F
- Aggression
- Racing heartbeat
- Rapid shallow breathing
- Cessation of sweating
- Confusion
- Nausea/ vomiting
- Red flushed skin
- Headache
- Extremely thirsty
- Disorientated, dizzy, slurred speech.
- Convulsions, seizures, coma

Call for emergency medical assistance. While waiting for assistance treat the patient the same as for heat exhaustion.

Hypothermia

Extreme cold weather or long periods of time exposed to cold weather especially in windy conditions or with inadequate clothing can cause Hypothermia.

Symptoms of Hypothermia

- Feeling cold and uncontrollable shivering. (shivering may stop as the person progresses to server hypothermia).

- Skin feels cold and looks pale.

- Drowsiness, slurred speech, unsteady gait.

- Confusion, tiredness, gradual loss of motor skills.

- Slowed heart rate and breathing, dilated pupils.

- As the symptoms may develop gradually, you may be unaware you are developing Hypothermia.

- Even though a person with hypothermia's body core temperature is dropping rapidly they may begin to feel extremely hot and want to shed their clothing. This will only exacerbate the problem.

Treatment of Hypothermia

- Call for emergency medical attention.

- Move the person out of the cold and remove any wet clothing.

- Warm the person especially on the chest, head, and neck areas. Use warm blankets, towels wrapped with hot water bottles or skin to skin contact. Do not massage the skin or apply heat directly using a heat lamp.

- Keep the person calm and still.

- Give warm fluids. Do not give alcohol.

Nosebleed

Most nosebleed are not serious and are easily managed. However, if you have a nosebleed that will not stop bleeding there may be an underlying cause and you should seek medical attention.

Treatment for a nosebleed

- Have the person sit upright and lean slightly forward to avoid swallowing blood. Breathe through the mouth.

- Have person pitch their nose below the bridge (bony part) with their thumb and index finger for 5-10 minutes to help stop the bleeding.

- Spit out any blood that enters your mouth.

- An ice pack can be placed on the person's forehead and back of the neck especially if the nosebleed is due to hot weather.

- If bleeding restarts, pinch nose again for 5-10 minutes.

- If bleeding will not stop after 20-30 minutes, or a broken nose is suspected, then seek medical attention.

Once bleeding has stopped:

- Do not blow or pick at your nose as it may restart the bleeding.

- Do not do any strenuous activity for 24 hours.

- Do not pack the nostrils with tissue or cotton wool.

Wounds

A wound is any damage or break in the surface of the skin and can be either Acute or Chronic (**www.healthywa.wa.gov.au**).

Acute wounds can include minor cuts, lacerations, abrasions, and bites.

Chronic wounds are wounds that are slow to heal such as ulcers.

Infection

It is important when dealing with wounds to monitor for infection. If infection is suspected, emergency medical assistance should be sought. Signs of infection are:

- redness
- pain
- swelling
- odour
- fever
- heat
- weeping fluid or pus from wound.

Treatment for wounds

- Apply gentle pressure with a clean towel or cloth to help control the bleeding.

- Wash your hands well prior to cleaning and dressing the wound to help stop contamination/infection.

- Rinse the wound with clean water to remove any blood, dirt etc. Then dry the surrounding skin with a clean towel.

- Replace any skin flaps that is still attached using a clean, moist cotton bud/Q-tip.

- Apply a thin layer of antibiotic cream and cover wound with a clean non-stick dressing then bandage in place.

- Change the bandage each day or when it becomes wet or dirty to help prevent infection.

Seek emergency medical attention if:

The wound will not stop bleeding.

There are signs of infection.

You have another injury or risk of further injury.

You have an underlying condition such as diabetes.

The wound is deep or will not heal.

The wound has dirt, glass, or other foreign object that you cannot remove.

Shock

Shock can be caused by many circumstances including loss of blood, allergic reaction, trauma, heatstroke, burns, infection and burns.

When in shock a person's vital organs such as their heart and brain are not getting enough oxygen. This can be life-threatening if not treated.

Symptoms of shock

- Weak rapid pulse
- Cold, Clammy skin
- Sweating
- Nausea
- Thirst
- Confusion
- Dizziness
- Gasping for air
- Loss of consciousness.

Treatment for shock

Call for emergency medical assistance. Do not leave person unattended.

Have the person lay on their back with their feet elevated unless they have a snakebite or broken leg.

Try to keep the person calm. Reassure them.

Cover their shoulders with a blanket, loosen any tight clothing.

Treat any wound or burn if possible.

Give small frequent sips of water to person who does not have abdominal injury.

Place person in the recovery position if they have trouble breathing, become unconscious or likely to vomit.

Commence CPR if person stops breathing.

(healthywa.wa.gov.au)

Snake bite

Treat all snake bites as potentially deadly. Get urgent emergency medical attention as soon as possible.

Ask the person to remember a description of the snake that bit them if possible as this can aid in identification. Do not try to catch the snake!

Treatment of snake bite

- While waiting for medical assistance, keep the person calm and sitting still. Make a note of the time.

- Do not wash, squeeze, or puncture the bite site.

- Do not try and *suck out* the venom.

- Apply a pressure immobilization bandage.

- Remove any jewellery on the limb in case of swelling.

- Do not allow victim to walk unless there is no other choice.

How to apply a pressure immobilisation bandage to a leg

- Apply a broad pressure bandage from below the bite site, over the bite site and above as high as possible.
- Wrap the bandage tightly. The person should remain as still as possible to help stop the flow of venom into the blood.

- Apply a splint firmly to the leg if possible, to help immobilise the leg.

Sprain

A sprain or strain is an injury to the tendons or muscles. They can be quite painful and will take some time to fully heal.

Treatment of a sprain

- Help person sit or lie down. Elevate injured limb and rest on pillows or towels.

- Apply a cold ice or gel pack to the area for 10-15 minutes.

- Use over the counter pain relief and anti-inflammatories to help with any swelling and pain management.

- Place a compression bandage over the sprained area if possible and keep elevated.

- Apply ice /cold pack to the injured area for 0-15 minutes four times a day for the next four days. If improvement is not made after 4 days, or a fever develops seek medical assistance.

- Crutches or a splint may be needed for the first few days of recovery. Try not to walk on or use the limb too often.

Chapter Thirty-three

Make your own supplies.

Hand sanitiser.

The best way to sanitize your hands is with soap and running water. Hand sanitizer is also a good way to sanitize, especially if you are away from home, however, hand sanitizer is usually one of the first items to become unavailable in stores during a public health crisis. You can make your own sanitizer, however, be sure to have at least 70% alcohol or the sanitizer will not be strong enough to kill bacteria and viruses. Do not use whiskey, vodka etc. as it is not strong enough.

Some people may have reactions to hand sanitizer so always do a patch test first by testing on a small area of skin such as your wrist before using.

Gel recipe

Ingredients
1/3 cup Glycerine or Aloe Vera Gel
2/3 cup 99% Rubbing Alcohol (isopropyl alcohol) 8-
10 drops tee tree, lemon, peppermint, or lavender
essential oil (or your favourite)
Funnel
Pump or squeeze bottle/s
Jug for mixing

Instructions

Make sure you have clean hands before starting.
Sanitize bottles, jug, and funnel by washing in hot
water.

Mix all ingredients and pour into bottles. The World
Health Organisation recommends you let your
concoction sit for 72 hours before using to ensure
any bacterial introduced during the mixing process
is killed.

**https://www.who.int/gpsc/5may/Guide_to_Loca
l_Production.pdf**

Spray recipe

Ingredients

340 ml/12 oz Isopropyl alcohol
2 Tablespoons Glycerol or glycerine
1 Tablespoon Hydrogen peroxide
85 ml/3 oz Distilled water (or tap water boiled and cooled)
Mixing jug.
Funnel
Spray bottles

Instructions

Sanitize jug, funnel, and spray bottle by washing in hot water.

Mix alcohol, glycerol (this helps to stop the alcohol from drying your hands out, however, you can make the mixture without it, just moisturize your hands afterwards), hydrogen peroxide and water. Pour into spray bottles.

This mixture can also be used on a paper towel to use as a wipe.

Oral rehydration preparation

While children, the sick and elderly are most at risk of dehydration, anyone can suffer the effects of dehydration and it can even be fatal if severe enough and not treated. Most pharmacies have oral supplies of ready to use rehydration liquid or powder available, and a supply should be kept in your medical first aid kit at home. If you are not able to go to a pharmacy because you are in a lockdown/isolation situation, you can make your own oral rehydration preparation using goods you will have in your home.

Ingredients

4 Tablespoons lemon juice
½ cup honey
½ teaspoon salt
1 Litre/1000 ml/ 1-quart warm water

Instructions

Mix all ingredients together and sip slowly to replenish the body's electrolyte balance.

Disinfectant solution

When you need to sanitise or disinfect surfaces around your home you can make your own disinfectant using simple products. Keep away from carpets and material as staining/ whitening may occur. Wear gloves when using.

Mix 1-part household bleach to 9-parts water. Wipe surface using solution. If food is to be prepared on the area, wipe with water afterwards.

Or

Spray surface with 3% hydrogen peroxide (available from pharmacists) followed by white vinegar. Keep these two ingredients in separate bottles away from the light.

Use to wipe down doorknobs, computer keyboards, tv remotes, children's toys, countertops, and anything else that needs disinfecting.

Gel Pack

A gel pack is a great way to relieve sore, aching muscles and to help reduce pain and swelling.

Ingredients

Ziplock plastic sandwich bag.
1 ½ cups water.
½ cup rubbing alcohol.

Instructions

Mix the water and rubbing alcohol inside the plastic bag and seal shut tightly. Do not completely fill the bag.

Freeze the bag for 4 hours.

The mixture will become cold and slushy but not completely frozen.

To use the gel pack, wrap a cloth or towel around it and apply to the sore/ swollen muscle. You can refreeze the pack when it is no longer cold.

Saline Spray

Having a blocked nose can be extremely annoying making it difficult to sleep. Using a saline spray to help clear out the nasal cavity can give you some relief from the congestion and make it easier to breath. If you do not have a saline spray at home, you can make one yourself with a few simple ingredients you will have in the kitchen.

Ingredients

Non iodised table or sea salt.

Distilled water. If you do not have distilled water use 1 cup of tap water boiled for 10 minutes, then cooled.

Baking Soda.

Saucepan

Small sterile bottle or bulb syringe.

Instructions

Add ¼ teaspoon of salt to 1 cup of distilled or boiled, cooled tap water.

Add a pinch of baking soda.

Pour water mixture into the sterile bottle or bulb syringe.

Close one nostril with your finger, then squirt the liquid three times into the other cavity. Repeat on the other side. Gentle blow nose.

This will help to moisturise and relieve dry/swollen nasal passages.

Substitutes for toothpaste, shampoo, and fire-starters.

Shampoo substitute

Ingredients

2 empty shampoo bottles or similar.
½ cup baking soda
1 ¼ cups water
¼ cup apple cider vinegar
Few drops of lavender oil or other fragrance.

Instructions

In one bottle mix the baking soda and ½ cup of water. Shake well.
In the other bottle mix the apple cider vinegar, ¾ cup of water and fragrance if required.

To use, wet your hair thoroughly then rub your hair and scalp with some of the baking soda mixture. Rinse with plain water.
Then rinse hair with some of the apple cider vinegar solution.

Toothpaste substitute

Ingredients

Baking soda.
Tap or bottled water.

Instructions

A quite simple substitute for toothpaste is to apply some baking soda to your toothbrush or finger if you don't have a toothbrush! Clean teeth as you would normally then, rinse well with fresh water.
It doesn't taste wonderful; however, it will keep your teeth clean and may even help to whiten them!

Firestarter substitute

Ingredients

10 cotton balls.
Petroleum jelly (Vaseline).
Bottle or jar with lid.
Label or permanent marker.

Instructions

Smear petroleum jelly over each cotton ball.
Label a bottle or jar *fire starters* and add the cotton balls. Close lid.

When you need to start a fire, place one or two of the cotton balls under your tinder and light with a long match or lighter.
The petroleum jelly will catch fire just like a fire starter!

Remember to take care when using fire starters and always supervise children and pets around a fire. Never leave a fire unattended.

Chapter Thirty-four

Using Herbs for Household Use

Herbs can be used as both a source of nourishment and for common household uses. Having a small herb garden in your yard can be greatly beneficial. Most herbs do not need a lot of space to grow and many can be grown in pots and even in containers on windowsills.

Herbs that are easy to grow include:
Lavender
Rosemary
Mint
Parsley
Peppermint
Oregano

Lavender and peppermint are particularly useful herbs for use as insect repellents.

Ants – Peppermint
Fleas – Lavender
Mosquitoes – Peppermint
Flies - - Lavender
Moths – Lavender

Moth Repellent Sachets

Ingredients

1/3 cup dried peppermint leaves
1/3 cup dried lavender flowers
3 drops of Lavender essential oil.
Cotton or muslin sachet

Instructions

Mix ingredients together in a bowl crushing the flowers a little to release their aroma.

Then, place the mixture in a cotton or muslin sachet and tie at the top. Place the sachet in your clothing wardrobe, kitchen pantry or with your food storage supplies to help keep out the moths.

They will also aid in keeping silverfish and ants away.

Kids love helping to make these so get them involved too. They can place them by their pillows or in their clothing drawers.

(The good living guide)

Herbal steam for sinus relief

Ingredients

1 teaspoon dried Chamomile flowers
1 teaspoon dried Rosemary leaf
1 teaspoon dried Peppermint leaf
4 drops of Eucalyptus oil

Instructions

Boil water and pour into a large plastic basin or bowl.

Add the herbs and let sit for 5 minutes.

Add the Eucalyptus oil.

Sit at a table and place your head over the bowl (be careful not to burn yourself with the hot water or steam. Cover your head with a dish cloth/tea towel, close your eyes and inhale the vapours.
The vapours will help to open the sinus passages making it easier to breath.

Mustard Foot Bath

Ingredients

2 Tablespoons of mustard powder or crushed mustard seeds
1 Tablespoon grated ginger
5 drops eucalyptus oil.
Warm water in a foot bath or bucket

Instructions

Add ingredients to warm water and soak feet in the *foot bath*. Good for aching muscles and to warm up cold feet.

Other essential oils such as lavender can be used instead of the eucalyptus oil if preferred.

Sunburn Relief Spray

Ingredients

50 mls Aloe Vera Gel
10 drops of Lavender Oil
3 drops of Peppermint oil.
10 mls distilled water

Instructions

Place all ingredients in a spray bottle and shake well.

Spray liberally and frequently onto sunburnt area. For severe sunburn seek medical attention.

If you have sensitive skin do a patch test first by spraying the gel on a small area of skin such as the inside of the wrist and wait for a few hours.

Other Household Products

Apple Cider Vinegar

Apple cider vinegar can be a very useful household product and can be used in a number of applications.

Sunburn
To ease mild sunburn, soak a cloth in a solution of one part vinegar and eight parts water. Apply gently to the sunburnt skin.

Sore throat
Gargle with ½ teaspoon of apple cider vinegar in 250 mls warm water to help kill bacteria.

Skin inflammation
Apple cider vinegar can help reduce skin inflammation and itching. Soak a cloth in one part vinegar and 4 parts cool water and apply to the inflamed area for 10 minutes twice a day.

Rubbing Alcohol

Rubbing alcohol is a useful antiseptic for sterilizing tweezers, needles and other medical instruments.
It can also be used on insect bites and athletes' foot to help with healing.

Epsom Salts

Sore Feet
Epsom salts or Magnesium Sulphate can be used to help relieve aching feet by dissolving ½ cup in a foot bath.

Splinters
To help remove a splinter soak a cloth in a solution of Epsom salts and water and apply to the area with the splinter for several minutes or soak the area in the solution. Then, use clean tweezers to remove the splinter.

Slugs
Epsom salts can be sprinkled around the base of your plants to deter slugs from eating your plants.

Hydrogen Peroxide

A small amount of Hydrogen Peroxide in a 3% concentration can be placed on cuts to help prevent infection. Let the area dry, then apply a bandage.

Chapter Thirty-five

Backyard Self Sufficiency

If you want to take things a step further to being self-sufficient into the future some ideas, you may want to consider include:

Growing your own vegetable and herb garden.

For this you will need a spot with good soil or potting mix with 6 hours of sunlight a day, fertilizer and plenty or water. Easy to grow plants include lemons, tomatoes, capsicums, potatoes, lettuce, beans, mint, parsley, and rosemary.

Grow an indoor garden.

For those households without a backyard or limited space, a small window garden, table that sits in the sunshine or balcony can be used.

Obviously, you won't be able to grow vegetables that need a lot of space however, many plants and herbs such as parsley, basil, mint, oregano, peppers, cherry tomatoes, and lettuce grow well in pots. Make sure they are well drained and have adequate sunshine. Growing a garden like this can be great fun for the kids too!

Water tank.

For a water tank to work properly it will need a roof to attach to for rainwater runoff. The water can then be used to water your garden or drink if sanitized first.

Solar Power.

Solar power panels can be added to your house to supplement your electricity supply and you may even be able to sell some back to your electrical supplier. There are many solar power companies available now offering deals on adding solar power to your house, however, these vary in quality so do your research before purchasing.

Chicken Coop.

A great way to have a fresh supply of eggs is to keep chickens in your back yard. They will need enough space to roam and a covered nesting area to sleep. You will also need to provide them with hay for bedding, pellets and vegetable scraps for food, plus drinking water.

Not all councils and areas allow chickens especially in city areas, so you will need to check your local rules and guidelines before purchasing any poultry. For example, roosters are usually not allowed in suburban areas.

Make your own composter.

You can build an outdoor composter using a 110 litre /30-gallon barrel. First drill some holes in the bottom for drainage, then layer 6 inches/ 100 cm of small sticks in the bottom for air circulation. Next layer grass cuttings and kitchen waste (vegetable and fruit scraps, eggshells, tea, and coffee grounds. No meat or dairy products.)
Keep the contents moist and roll the barrel around every few days to keep it aerated.
Once the barrel is full it will take approximately 6 weeks to decompose into rich soil for your garden. If you have two compost barrels working you can alternate between them.

Learn First Aid

Every adult in your household and even older children should have some basic first aid training including how to administer CRP (cardiopulmonary resuscitation). First Aid courses are available through the red cross and St Johns Ambulance offices.

Chapter Thirty-six

Evacuate/Relocate.

Sometimes for the safety of your family you have no other choice but to evacuate your home and relocate. The period of evacuation could be for a short while for example, during a power outage in a heatwave/ice storm, or it could be for a longer period- think Hurricane Katrina.

Evacuating your home can be stressful. What do I take? What do I leave behind? Will we have enough time? If your family has an evacuation/relocation plan made in advance everyone will know what they are supposed to be doing helping to keep your stress levels and blood pressure much lower!

When you evacuate take your emergency kit and relocation kit with you. See the appendices at the back of the book for examples of an emergency kit and relocation kit.

When making your evacuation plan, give every member of your household a job/responsibility. This will take the pressure off you to do and remember everything. Even young children can have a *job* such as remembering to pack their favourite blanket/toy (make a quick check on this before you leave!)

Some of the things to include in your evacuation plan are:

- Turning off the electricity, gas, and water.

- Locking doors and windows.

- What to do with your pets.

- Taking valuables with you (this is an individual choice whether it be money, jewellery, trophies, awards, or photo albums).

- Turn off computers, television, and other electronics.

- Prepare your car, does it have enough petrol/gas to get where you are going. Good tyres etc.

- Who will you tell where you are going and when you are leaving?

- Do you have food and water to take with you?

- What special items are you taking with you for the elderly, babies, pregnant women, disabled sick etc?

- What prescription medications will you need to take with you?

- Do you have a car charger for your phone and or computer so you can charge them while you are driving? This way you can keep in contact with people.

- And lastly where are you going? Do you have a map or GPS on how to get there? Roads may be blocked, inaccessible or jammed with traffic. Do you have an alternate route planned?

Do you know how to signal for help if you become stranded?

- Lift the boot/trunk and bonnet/hood of your car to signal you need help.

- Blowing on a whistle three times, wait for a few minutes and repeat.

- If the sun is out, use a mirror or shiny object such as aluminium foil or the bottom of a soft drink can to signal SOS. Three short flashes, three long flashes, three short flashes.
- The same can be done at night-time with a flashlight/torch.

- Use rocks, sticks branches or any other material to spell our SOS on the ground or your car roof.

Chapter Thirty-seven

After a Disaster

Food Supplies after a flood, hurricane, or cyclone

Do not eat any food that has had any contact with floodwater as it can harbour dangerous pathogens. Dry food is particularly vulnerable as it is susceptible to mould and fungus.

Use gloves when handling any food that may have spoiled or be contaminated and wash your hands in warm soapy water.

If cans or jars of food are waterproof and undamaged, they can still be used. Remove the labels and wash the containers in hot, soapy water.

Make a solution of 1 Tablespoon of bleach to 4.5 Litres/1 gallon and immerse the tins for 15 minutes. Remove the tins and air dry for one hour before re labelling. Consume as usual, however, these should be used as soon as possible and not stored for a length of time.
https://www.cdc.gov

Any cooking and eating utensils, plates, bowls etc. that have come into contact with flood water must also be sanitized.

After the power is restored

Check your food for safety.
If a power outage is less than 4 hours most of your food in your refrigerator should be fine as long as the door was kept closed. Perishable foods such as dairy products, lunch meats and seafood should be discarded.

Any thawed meat should be cooked immediately. If the power outage has been for an extended period or you are unsure, throw the meat away.

Check each package individually as smaller packets will thaw more quickly than larger ones. Food may look fine but harbour bacteria that can cause deadly food borne illnesses.

Pets

Pets can find disasters such as fire, storms, cyclones, and floods very stressful and will need reassurance. This is particularly true if their usual surroundings are changed because of flood or fire, for example.

If you are returning to your home after an emergency or disaster, ensure you release your pet in an enclosed space to get them used to their surroundings before letting them roam freely outside. Distressed animals may become disorientated, frightened or aggressive. They may also try to run away.

Give them lots of encouragement and attention.

Your Wellbeing

Experiencing a disaster or emergency can be a frightening, overwhelming, and stressful experience. It can be both physically and mentally draining especially if you have children, or others with special needs to also care for.

When disasters are unexpected or significant, they can be disruptive to your life and leave you and your family feeling unsettled and anxious for a while after the event.

The Department of Fire and Emergency services suggests that after an emergency it is common to feel depression, fatigue, anger, sadness and have nightmares. You may also continually think about the event, have trouble making decisions or concentrating, feel stressed, irritable, teary, overwhelmed and have disturbed sleep.

Remember you have been through an extremely stressful event and it is alright to feel emotional. If you find you do not return to your usual routine within a few weeks or you feel unable to cope, you should seek professional help.

Children's' wellbeing

Children can also suffer from stress following an emergency or disaster especially if it was frightening or unexpected. Understand and recognise your child's responses. They may be irritable, unable to sleep, teary, clingy, angry or revert to old behaviours such as bed wetting or sucking their thumb.

Give your children support and comfort and let them know you are there to talk with them about what happened, their feelings, and thoughts if they wish to. Children may also find it beneficial to draw or write about their experience.

Seek medical assistance if your child becomes withdraw, depressed or shows other behaviours that concern you.

Positive ways help your family cope after a disaster.

Avoid too many stimulants such as coffee, cigarettes, and energy drinks. Your sleep may already be affected, and caffeine will not help the situation.

Drink lots of water and try to eat regular, healthy meals together as a family.

Open discussion about the disaster if people feel the need to talk about it. Remember, some people may not wish to talk about the event or situation at all.

Get lots of sleep or at least rest if you cannot sleep.

Spend time talking to and being with people you care about. If children cannot see their friends, let them skype, text or facetime.

Avoid drinking too much alcohol. It may seem like a way to cope, however; it may create more problems.

Try to return to a daily routine of work, school, exercise or whatever your normal family daily routine is even if it is a limited version.

If your community has been affected by the disaster, become involved in community activities to help rebuild your area.

Focus on making daily decisions rather than large major ones. This will help you to feel in control of your life again.

Restock your emergency kit, first aid kit, relocation kit, pet kit etc.

Ask for support from family, friends, counsellors, doctors or other professionals if you need it.

Call your doctor, Crisis Care, Lifeline or the Good Samaritans in your area if you feel you cannot cope, are unable to carry out your normal routines, feel hopeless or are thinking of harming yourself or anyone else.

Chapter Thirty-eight

Easy Recipes

Chicken and vegetable Ramen noodles

Ingredients

• 2 packets of ramen or two-minute noodles. (other instant type noodles can also be used) Flavour sachet is not needed.
• 1 Tablespoon oil
• 2 garlic cloves crushed (garlic granules can also be used)
• ½ sliced onion
• 200 g chicken thighs cut into small pieces. (remove for a vegetarian version)

- 1 ¼ cups of water
- 1 small red capsicum/bell pepper (frozen can be used)
- 2 cups cabbage finely sliced.

Sauce

- 1 Tablespoon soy sauce
- 1 Tablespoon Oyster sauce
- 2 teaspoons Hoisin sauce
- 1 Tablespoon Mirin

Instructions

Mix sauce ingredient together.

Heat oil in a wok or frypan over high heat. Add onion and garlic and cook until starting to go golden.
Be careful they don't burn.

Add chicken and cook until outside is white in colour.
Add sauce mixture and cook for one minute or until chicken is caramelized.
Add cabbage and capsicum and cook for one minute.

Push the chicken and vegetable mixture to one side of the frypan and add water into the space. Place dried noodles into the water, and simmer for one minute.

Toss noodle mixture through the vegetables and sauce until coated. Add chopped cabbage. Fold though for one minute and serve immediately.

Beef and Bean Enchiladas or Bean Enchiladas

Note: any frozen vegetables, beans, lentils, or chicken mince can be added or substituted for beef the filling.

<u>Ingredients</u>

- 8 tortillas or burrito wraps
- 1.5 cups cheese (tasty, cheddar or mozzarella)

Enchilada Sauce
- 2 Tablespoons olive oil
- 3 Tablespoons flour
- 2 cups (500 mls) chicken stock or vegetable if making vegetarian.
- 1 ½ cups tomato passata
- Salt and pepper to season

Spice   Mix
combine
- 1 Teaspoon onion powder
- 1 Teaspoon garlic powder
- 1 Tablespoon cumin powder, paprika and dried oregano.

Filling
- 1 Tablespoon olive oil
- 2 garlic cloves crushed.
- 1 brown onion finely chopped (dried onion flakes or frozen onion can also be used)

- 500 g minced beef or 1 can refried beans.
- 1 tin red kidney beans drained.

Instructions

Make enchilada sauce.

Heat oil in saucepan over medium heat, add flour and mix to a paste, cook for one minute, stirring continuously.

Add ½ cup chicken or vegetable stock and whisk until smooth. Slowly add remaining stock, passata, salt, pepper and two tablespoons of spice mix.

Increase heat slightly, continue to stir until sauce thickens.

Remove from stove.

Make the filling

Preheat oven to 180 C/ 350 F.

Heat oil in frypan over high heat, add garlic and onion and cook for 2 minutes.
Add beef and cook for 2 minutes, add remaining spice mix, and cook until browned. Add red kidney beans, salt, and pepper and ¼ cup of enchilada sauce. Cook for 2 minutes then remove from heat.

Construct Enchiladas

Grease baking dish.

Place filling in each tortilla, roll up then place in baking dish seam side down. Pour sauce over enchiladas and top with cheese.

Bake in oven for 10 minutes covered with aluminium foil, then 10 minutes uncovered.

Serve hot with a salad or vegetables.

One pot cauliflower, chicken, and rice.

Ingredients

- 2 Tablespoons butter
- 1 Tablespoon olive oil
- 1 brown onion finely chopped (dried onion flakes or frozen onion can also be used)
- 2 garlic cloves crushed (garlic granules can also be used)
- 500 g chicken thigh cut into small pieces.
- 2 ½ Tablespoons of flour or cornflour
- 2 cups milk (fresh or long life)
- 2 cups of chicken stock (or use stock cubes in water)
- 1 ¼ cups white rice uncooked (long grain, jasmine or basmati)
- 1 teaspoon dried thyme (or other preferred herb)
- Salt and pepper
- ½ head cauliflower cut into florets (broccoli can also be used, or frozen vegetables thawed and drained of water)
- 2 cups grated cheese (mozzarella, tasty or cheddar)

Instructions

Melt butter and oil in a pot over high heat, add onion and garlic and cook for one minute. Add chicken and cook until white in colour. Turn heat down to medium, add flour and stir for one minute. Slowly add milk to flour mixture, stir continuously until thickened.

Add stock, rice, herbs, salt, and pepper. Bring to a simmer then turn down heat, cover and cook for twelve minutes.

Add cauliflower and push into rice mixture until covered. Cover again and cook for a further 3 minutes until cauliflower is just cooked.

Remove lid and stir through half the cheese. Top with remaining cheese and grill.

Serve hot.

Creamy chicken fettuccine

Ingredients

- 300 g fettuccine or other dried pasta
- 2 Tablespoons butter
- 2 chicken breasts cut in half length ways.
- Salt and pepper
- 2 garlic cloves crushed or garlic granules.
- ½ cup dry white wine or extra chicken stock
- ½ cup chicken stock
- 1 ¼ cups thickened cream.
- ¾ cup finely grated parmesan
- 70 g baby spinach
- 100 g sundried tomatoes if available
-

Instructions

Sprinkle chicken with salt and pepper on both sides. Melt butter in fry pan over high heat. Add chicken and cook for 2 minutes on each side until golden coloured. Remove chicken from pan, rest for a few minutes, then shred with 2 forks. Cook pasta in large pot of salted boiling water. Drain pasta keeping one cup of the liquid to one side.

Make sauce by adding remaining butter and oil to frypan and melting over a medium heat. Add garlic and cook until golden, add wine. Simmer rapidly stirring.

Add chicken stock, cream, parmesan cheese and tomatoes. Simmer for 3-5 minutes stirring until sauce reduces and thickens. Add pasta to sauce, tossing to coat.

Add some of the reserved pasta liquid if the sauce is too thick.

Serve hot with added grated parmesan if desired.

Creamy tuna pasta bake

Ingredients

- 350 g penne pasta or other pasta
- 3 Tablespoons butter
- 3 garlic cloves crushed.
- 4 Tablespoons flour
- 4 cups milk (long life milk can be used)
- 2 Teaspoons chicken or vegetable stock powder
- 1/2 cup parmesan cheese finely grated.
- ½ Teaspoon of mustard powder
- ½ Teaspoon onion powder
- ½ Teaspoon garlic powder
- 425 g canned tuna drained (salmon can also be used)
- 400 g tinned corn drained (other tinned vegetables such as peas can be used)

Topping
- 1 ½ Tablespoons butter melted.
- 1/2 cup panko breadcrumbs (other breadcrumbs may also be used)
- ¼ cup grated parmesan cheese
- ¼ Teaspoon salt

Instructions

Preheat oven to 180° C/ 356 F. Mix together topping ingredients and put to one side.
Cook pasta in a pot of salted boiling water until almost cooked then drain. Return to pot.

Make white sauce by melting butter in a large pot over medium heat, add garlic and cook until golden. Add flour and whisk. Gradually pour in milk. Add stock powder, mustard, onion, and garlic powder. Turn down heat and cook until sauce thickens. Whisk continuously to ensure sauce does not burn. Remove from stove and stir in parmesan.

Add tuna into pasta and flake into large chunks with fork, add corn or other vegetable and pour over sauce stir through gently. Transfer mixture to a baking dish and top with crunchy topping.

Bake for 25 minutes or until top is golden.

Chicken with Cashew nuts

Ingredients

- 500 g chicken thigh/breast or tenders cut into small pieces or strips.
- 2 Tablespoons peanut oil (vegetable oil can also be used)
- 2 garlic cloves crushed or garlic granules.
- ½ onion chopped (white or brown)
- 1 green or red capsicum / bell pepper chopped into 2 cm pieces.
- 6 Tablespoons water
- ¾ cup roasted unsalted cashews.

Sauce
- 1 Tablespoon corn flour/corn-starch
- 3 Teaspoons soy sauce
- 3 Tablespoons Chinese cooking wine or Mirin
- 3 Tablespoons oyster sauce
- 2 Teaspoons sesame oil

Instructions

Make sauce by mixing corn flour and soy sauce until there are no lumps. Add remaining sauce ingredients. Use two tablespoons of the mixture to coat the chicken. Set aside for 10 minutes to marinate.

Heat oil over high heat in a wok or frypan, add garlic and onion and cook for one minute. Add chicken. Cook for two minutes then add the capsicum and cook for a further minute.
Next add the sauce mix and water. Bring to a simmer and cook until sauce thickens. Stir through cashews.

Serve with rice, Hokkien noodles or cauliflower rice.

Chilli con carne

Ingredients

- 1 Tablespoon olive oil
- 3 garlic cloves crushed (dried garlic can also be used)
- 1 onion diced (dried onion flakes or frozen onion can also be used)
- 1 red capsicum/ bell pepper diced (frozen can be used)
- 500 g beef mince / ground beef
- 3 Tablespoons tomato paste
- 800 g can crushed tomato.
- 420 g can red kidney beans drained (other beans can also be used)
- Pinch of salt

For a **vegetarian option** remove mince and add extra beans and tinned corn. Mince substitute and mushrooms can also be added.

Spice mix

3 teaspoons of Mexican chilli powder **or**

- 1 Teaspoon cayenne pepper
- 1 Teaspoon paprika powder
- 1 Teaspoons cumin powder
- 1 Teaspoons garlic powder
- 1 Teaspoons onion powder

To serve
Rice or corn chips or baked potato
Grated cheese, sour cream

Instructions

Heat oil in a frypan over medium high heat. Add garlic and onion, cook for 1 minute. Add capsicum and cook until onion is translucent. Increase heat and add mince. Cook until brown.

Add spice mix, tomato paste and tinned tomato. Simmer stirring occasionally for 10 minutes.

Serve over rice, ladle into bowls, and serve with corn chips, stir through pasta, or use to stuff baked potatoes. The chilli can also be frozen for later use.

Curry cauliflower soup

Ingredients

- 1 cauliflower head cut into florets.
- 200 g potatoes peeled and chopped.
- 1 brown onion sliced into rings.
- 2 cloves garlic unpeeled (garlic granules may be used instead and added with other spices)
- 1 Teaspoon ground cumin
- 1 Teaspoon ground coriander
- 2 Teaspoons curry powder
- Salt and pepper
- ¼ cup olive oil
- 4 cups vegetable stock (or water)
- ½ cup milk (long life milk or substitute can be used)
- 1 ½ cups finely grated parmesan cheese

Instructions

Pre heat oven to 220 C

Place cauliflower, garlic cloves with skin on, potato and onion on lined baking tray. Drizzle with olive oil. Roast for 25 minutes or until vegetables are tender.

Place vegetables and peeled garlic into a food processor with two cups of stock and blend until a smooth puree.

Transfer puree to a large pot, add remaining stock and milk. Add spices and bring to the boil. Stir in parmesan and season with salt and pepper.

Serve hot with crusty bread.

Soup can be frozen for later use.

Baked Spaghetti

Ingredients

- 500 g spaghetti
- 8 – 10 slices Swiss cheese or other cheese.
- 2 cups (200 g) mozzarella cheese grated.

Bolognese sauce

- 2 Tablespoons olive oil.
- 3 garlic cloves minced.
- 1 onion chopped.
- 1 carrot finely diced (mix of tinned peas carrots and corn can also be used).
- 1 stick celery finely diced (optional).
- 750 g beef mince/ground beef.
- 3/4 cup (185 ml) dry red wine (beef or vegetable stock may be substituted).
- Two tins crushed tomato.
- ¼ cup tomato paste.
- 2 Teaspoons Worcestershire sauce.
- 3 dried bay leaves.
- ½ Teaspoon oregano.
- ½ teaspoon thyme.
- ½ teaspoon garlic granules.
- Salt and pepper.

Vegetarian option remove mince and add red kidney beans or other tinned drained beans.

Instructions

Pre heat oven to 180 C /356 F
Heat oil in a frypan over medium high heat, add garlic and onion and cook until translucent. Add celery and carrot. Cook for 3 minutes. Turn up heat, add mince and cook until brown. Add wine (or stock) and spices and simmer for two minutes. Add Worcester sauce, tomato paste and tinned tomato and stir through. Simmer over low heat for 20 minutes. Stirring occasionally so as not to burn bottom. Add water if too much sauce evaporates. Add salt and pepper.

While sauce is simmering, cook pasta in large pot of salted boiling water for 10 minutes or until al dente. Drain and return to pot. Add half the sauce and stir through.
Spread half the pasta in a casserole dish, layer with half remaining sauce. Top with cheese slices, then remaining pasta and remaining Sauce. Finish with grated mozzarella.
Cover loosely with foil and bake for 25 minutes. Remove foil and bake for a further 10 minutes. Cut slices with a knife and use a spatula to serve pieces like a lasagne!
Can be frozen and reheated in microwave.

Chicken or Salmon Yakitori Skewers

Ingredients

500 g chicken thigh fillets or salmon with skin removed.
¼ cup Mirin.
1/3 cup soy sauce.
2 Tablespoon honey.
2 Tablespoons sesame oil.
2 Teaspoons ginger finely grated.
1 clove garlic crushed.
2 red onions chopped into squares.
1 red capsicum cut into squares.
Olive oil.
Bamboo skewers (soak in cold water for 10 minutes before use to prevent burning).

Instructions

Whisk together mirin, soy sauce, honey, sesame oil, ginger, and garlic in a jug. Place chicken or fish in a shallow dish, pour half the marinade mixture over the top, cover with plastic wrap and chill for 30 minutes.

Cut capsicum and red onions into squares. Drain chicken or fish. Thread chicken (or fish), capsicum and onion alternately onto skewers.

Cook skewers in a frypan with a little olive oil or under a grill or on the BBQ. Turn regularly, brushing with remaining marinade. Cook for approximately 10 minutes or until cooked.
Serve with rice, pasta, or vegetables.

Shepard's Pie Parcels

Ingredients

- 1 Tablespoon olive oil.
- 1 brown onion finely chopped (dried onion flakes or frozen onion can also be used).
- 1 carrot finely chopped.
- 1/3 cup frozen peas.
- 300 g beef mince/ground beef.
- 1 Teaspoon dried oregano.
- 2 Tablespoons tomato paste.
- 1 ½ Tablespoons Worcestershire sauce.
- 1 Tablespoon flour.
- 4 sheets of frozen, thawed puff pastry.
- ½ cup grated cheddar, tasty or mozzarella cheese.
- 1 egg beaten.
- 4 large potatoes peeled and chopped.
- 2 Tablespoons milk.
  Tomato sauce to serve (optional).

Vegetarian version Remove beef and use drained tinned beans, chopped mushrooms or meat alternative instead.

Instructions

Pre-heat oven to 220 C/430 F, line two large baking trays with baking paper.
Heat oil in a large frypan over medium high heat. Cook onion and carrot for 5 minutes stirring. Add mince and oregano, cook until browned.

Add tomato paste, sauce and flour stir for 30 seconds then add ½ cup water, bring to the boil. Stir in peas, cook for 2 minutes until sauce thickens. Set aside to cool.
Cook potatoes in salted boiling water until soft, drain and add milk, mash until smooth.

Cut each pastry sheet in half to form 8 rectangles. Place 4 rectangles on prepared trays. Place mince, potato, and cheese on each rectangle. Top with remaining pastry. Using a fork, press edges of pastry together to seal.
Brush tops of pastry with beaten egg.

Bake in oven for 30 minutes or until golden.

Serve with tomato sauce if desired, steamed vegetables or salad.

Vegetarian Bolognese

Ingredients

500 g spaghetti or other pasta.
3 Tablespoon olive oil.
1 brown onion finely diced (onion flakes or frozen can also be used).
garlic crushed (garlic granules or powder can also be used).
1 carrot finely diced.
1 celery stick finely diced.
4 mushrooms chopped.
1 red capsicum finely diced (frozen can also be used).
420 g can lentils drained.
½ cup water.
1 Teaspoon oregano.
Pinch salt.

Instructions

Heat oil in a frypan and add onion and garlic, cook until translucent. Add carrot, celery, capsicum, and mushroom, cook until tender.

Stir in herbs, salt, tomato, and half cup of water, bring to the boil. Reduce heat and simmer for 10 minutes. Stir in lentils and cook for 2 minutes.

Cook spaghetti in salted boiling water until cooked.

Serve pasta topped with lentil Bolognese. Grated tasty or parmesan cheese can be sprinkled on top if desired.

This Bolognese sauce can also be used to stuff baked potatoes, just add sour cream and cheese on top and place in oven until potato is cooked.

One pot lemon chicken and rice

Ingredients

- 5 chicken thighs, skin on with bone Marinade
- 2 lemons
- 1 Tablespoon dried oregano
- 4 cloves garlic crushed (garlic granules can also be used)
- ½ teaspoon salt

Rice
- 1 ½ Tablespoons olive oil
- 1 small onion finely chopped.
- 1 cup long grain rice
- 1 ½ cups chicken stock
- 1 Tablespoon dried oregano
- ½ teaspoon salt
- Pepper

Instructions

Combine chicken and marinade ingredients in a zip lock bag and leave for 30 minutes.

Pre heat oven to 180 C 356 F

Remove chicken from marinade but retain marinade.

Heat ½ tablespoon of olive oil in a fry pan/skillet over medium high heat, cook chicken skin side down and cook until golden brown and turn and cook other side. Remove chicken and set aside. Wipe oil from frypan using a paper towel. Heat 1 Tablespoon of olive oil in frypan and add onion and cook until translucent.

Add remaining rice ingredients and remaining marinade. Simmer for 1 minute then add chicken pieces on top of rice. Place lid on top of frypan or use aluminium foil.

Bake in oven for 35 minutes. Remove lid and bake for another 10 minutes or until liquid is absorbed and rice is tender.

Remove from oven and rest for 5-10 minutes before serving. Garnish with zest of lemon and serve.

Spiced Lentils

Ingredients

- 1 ½ cups green lentils
- 1 ¾ cups chicken, beef, or vegetable stock
- 1 bay leaf
- ½ teaspoon cumin
- 1 garlic clove crushed (powder can also be used)
- 1 brown or white onion chopped finely.
- 1 tomato, chopped.
- 1 Tablespoon oil
- Salt and Pepper

Instructions

Rinse lentils in a mesh colander in cool water removing any stones.

In a pot over medium heat, warm the oil then add garlic, onion cumin and tomato. Sauté for 3 minutes or until onion turns translucent.

Add lentils and stock. Bring to the boil and cook for 20-30 minutes or until the lentils are tender.

Season with salt and pepper. Serve with rice or pasta.

Beef Jerky

Beef jerky is a good source of protein. The strips can be eaten as a snack or added to soup or stews. Soak overnight to rehydrate before adding them to the pot.

Ingredients

- ½ kilogram/ 2 pounds beef steak.
- cups beer
- 2 cups soy sauce.
- ½ cup Worcestershire sauce.
- 2 Tablespoons pepper.

Instructions

With a sharp knife slice the beef with the grain into 1 cm/ half inch slices.

In a bowl mix together beer, sauces, and pepper. Add beef to marinade coating the pieces well.

Cover and refrigerate for 8 hours or overnight.

Drain marinade and pat beef dry with paper towels.

Preheat oven to 100 degrees C/ 200 degrees F.

Grease oven tray with oil. Place strips of beef on the tray keeping them separated. Cook for 4 hours.

Remove from oven and let cool. The beef should be firm but chewy.

Pack in an airtight container.

Mexican beef and rice casserole

Ingredients

- 2 Tablespoon olive oil
- 1 onion finely chopped (onion flakes or frozen can also be used)
- 3 garlic cloves crushed (garlic granules can also be used)
- 500 g mince beef
- 1/3 cup tomato paste
- 1 ¼ cups white long-grain rice
- 2 1/2 cups chicken stock (stock cube and water can also be used)
- 400 g can corn kernels drained (frozen can also be used)
- 400 g red kidney beans drained (other beans can also be used)
- 1 capsicum/bell pepper diced (frozen can also be used)
- 1 cup spring onion chopped.
- 2 cups grated cheese.

Mexican spices

- ½ teaspoon cayenne pepper (optional)
- 2 teaspoons dried oregano
- 3 teaspoons cumin
- 3 teaspoons coriander
- 3 teaspoons onion powder

- 2 teaspoons paprika
- ½ teaspoon salt

Vegetarian version
Remove meat and add extra beans, meat alternative or cooked vegetarian sausages sliced.

Instructions

Heat oil in large pot over high heat, add garlic and onion and cook unit translucent.
Add beef and cook until brown. Add Mexican spices and cook for one minute.
Add tomato paste, stock, capsicum, and rice. Stir and cook for one minute.

Add corn and beans, cover and simmer over medium for 15 minutes. Remove lid, stir through spring onion and half cheese.
Smooth top and sprinkle with remaining cheese. Cover and leave for one minute for cheese to melt.

Serve.

Can be frozen and reheated in microwave.

Apple Pikelets /flapjacks

Ingredients

2 cups self-rising flour
2 Tablespoons sugar
1 cup milk (long life milk can be used)
1 egg or powdered eggs
Canned apple
Cinnamon powder
1 Tablespoon butter or margarine

Instructions

Sift flour into a bowl. Add sugar, egg and milk and whisk until lump free. Add cinnamon and drained tinned apple and stir through.

Heat butter or margarine in a frypan over medium heat. Add Tablespoons of mixture to the frypan and cook until bubbling then flip pikelets and cook on other side. Serve hot or cold.

Flour Tortillas

Ingredients
2 cups flour
Pinch salt
1 teaspoon baking powder
¼ cup vegetable oil
½ cup warm water

Instructions

Mix ingredients to from a dough. Cover with cling wrap or a dishcloth and let sit for 30 minutes in a warm spot.

Heat a frypan over medium heat. Divide dough into eight balls and roll each out into a circular shape on a floured board.

Fry in a dry pan until brown spots appear on the bottom. Flip the tortilla and cook on the other side until done.

While tortillas are hot fill with savoury filling such as beans, cheese, and salsa. Or sweet such as honey and fruit.

Making bread by hand

If you don't own a bread machine, you can make your own bread by hand. It is easy to do and gives you a workout at the same time!

Ingredients

350 ml lukewarm water
600 g bread flour
2 teaspoon dried yeast

Instructions

Preheat oven to 220 C / 430 F.

Place flour in a large mixing bowl. Add water and yeast and mix to form a dough.
Lightly flour your benchtop and knead the dough by hand vigorously until it is smooth and elastic.
Knead for 12 minutes.

Return dough to mixing bowl and cover with cling wrap or a dishcloth making sure there is enough room for the dough to rise. Place in a warm spot for 40 minutes.

Remove dough from bowl and knead lightly on a floured surface for two minutes to de-gas the dough.

Place in an oiled bread/loaf tin and bake dough in oven for 30- minutes or until golden.

To test whether bread is cooked, tap lightly. Loaf is cooked when you hear a hollow sound.

Allow to cool for a few minutes before slicing.

Once cool, bread can be placed in a plastic bag or container to keep fresh. Bread can also be frozen.

Appendices

Relocation Kit

Table 7 Family Relocation Kit

• A relocation kit is in addition to your emergency kit and is in case your family needs to evacuate in a hurry.
• Spare clothing including a hat.
• Secure, comfortable closed toe footwear (remember you may have to walk).
• Sleeping bags and bedding.
• Extra food and water.
• Pet leash/ carrier and other requirements.
• Personal documents.
• Insect repellent, sunscreen
• Rain gear other items.
• Waterproof matches

Bushfire Emergency Kit

Table 8 Bushfire Emergency Kit

Essentials
Prepare before bushfire season.
• Drinking water.
• Portable battery-operated radio.
• Waterproof torch or light.
• First Aid Kit.
• Candles/waterproof matches.
• Woollen blanket.
• Emergency contact numbers.
• Bushfire protective clothing –

Bushfire protective clothing includes loose fitting clothing made from natural fibres like wool, cotton, or denim. Long sleeved shirt, sturdy closed footwear, woollen or cotton socks, wide brimmed hat, gloves, fire protection goggles/glasses, face mask/respirator or wet cloth.

Important extras

Pack on the day

• Wallet/purse, keys, and phone with charger.
• Medication and toiletries.
• Important documents and valuables in a plastic bag.
• Spare clothing.
• Combination pocketknife.
• Pet needs.
• Specific requirements for your family members.

Pet Emergency Kit

Table 9 Pet Emergency Kit

• Non-perishable food for three weeks
• Drinkable water
• Food and water bowls
• Bedding/blankets
• Grooming equipment
• Couple of toys
• Litter/newspaper. Gloves and disinfectant
• Pet documents – licence, ownership etc
• Medications
• Pet identification and photo of pet
• Vet and Ranger number
• Lead/carrier

Bushfire Leave Early. Plan of Action

When will we leave?

Where will we go?

Who will we call to let them know we are leaving?

Which way will we go?

Route One

Alternate route

Where is our emergency kit located?

What will we take?

What is our back up plan if things go the way we planned?

Who will lock the house windows and doors?

Who will take the pets?

Pet Plan of Action

Pets name and age.

Name and phone number of veterinarian.

Name and phone number of Ranger.

Name and phone number of local animal welfare agency e.g., RSPCA.

Name of friend or relative able to look after pet.

Licence/registration number

Medications needed.

Adequate identification.

Photo of pet.
Organise food and water.

Organise bedding.

Organise sanitary equipment.

Leash or pet carrier

Food and water bowls

Other

Storm Plan of Action

Where is our emergency kit kept?

What outdoor items do we need to put away and secure?

Who will secure outdoor items?

Where do we turn off our supplies?

Electricity

Water

Gas

Who will be responsible for turning supplies off if needed?

What is our plan for our pets?

If we need to leave for a safer place where will we go?

Who will check windows and doors are locked before we leave?

What items will we take with us?

Emergency kit

Car keys

House keys

Phone

Other

Flood Plan of Action

Where is our emergency kit kept?

Where do we turn off our supplies?

Electricity

Water

Gas

Who will be responsible for turning supplies off if needed?

What is our plan for our pets?

If we need to leave for higher ground where will we go?

Who will check windows and doors are locked before we leave?

Who will empty refrigerator and Freezer?

What items will we take with us?

Emergency kit

Car keys

House keys

Phone

Other

Tornado Plan of Action

Where is our emergency kit kept?

Who will gather the emergency pack?

Where do we turn off our supplies?

Electricity

Gas

Who will be responsible for turning supplies off if needed?

Where will we shelter in the house during a tornado?

Who will gather blankets, mattress etc?

Who is responsible for the pets?

Who will close the window/storm shutters?

Who will secure outdoor/loose items if there is time?

Where will we meet after the tornado has passed?

Evacuation Plan of Action

Where is our emergency kit and relocation kit?

Who will collect these?

Where do we turn off the:
Water
Gas
Electricity

Who will turn these off?

Who will collect pets and pet kit?

Who will collect valuables?

Who will collect computer, phones, chargers?

Who will check the car for fuel etc?

Who will load car with supplies?

Who will we notify when we leave?

Who will do this?

Who will lock doors and windows?

Where are we evacuating to?

What is an alternative route?

Important Telephone Numbers

Table 10 Important Telephone Numbers

Police/Fire/Ambulance
Poison Control Centre
Emergency Management (state emergency services)
Veterinarian
Animal Rescue
Doctor
Specialist
Paediatrician

Children's school
Red Cross
Dentist
Gas company
Electrical Company
Water Services
Sewage Services
Repair Services
Insurance company
Neighbours
Family and Friends

First Aid Kit

- Plasters/band Aids of different sizes
- Bandages
- Pain relief such as paracetamol, ibuprofen, aspirin or similar
- Child pain relief
- Tweezers
- Scissors
- Ani Diarrhea medication
- Antihistamine
- Hydrocortisone cream
- Disposable Gloves
- Disposable masks
- Aloe Vera Gel
- Burn cream.
- Syringe
- Antiseptic cream or solution
- Gauze pads
- Petroleum Jelly
- Eyedrops
- Cotton swabs, balls, and Q-tips
- Safety Pins
- Thermometer
- Hand sanitizer
- Needle and thread
- Electrolyte solution (powder sachets)

- Family prescription medication e.g., asthma inhaler, diabetic medication, high blood pressure pill
- First Aid Manual
- Clove oil
- Toothache remedy
- Alcohol wipes
- Saline solution or eye wash
- Hydrogen peroxide or betadine
- Measuring spoon
- Bulb syringe
- Instant/disposable cold pack
- Roll of duct tape.
- Rescue blanket for shock
- Fire blanket
- Triangle bandage/sling
- Butterfly wound closures.
- Notepad and pen
- Snake bite pressure immobilization bandage.

- **Personal medications** such as asthma inhalers, insulin, heart tablets, high blood pressure tablets, blood thinners, anti-depressants, contraceptive pill, etc

Other medical supplies you may want to add include:

- Contact lenses and solution/ spare glasses.
- Cough suppressant

- throat lozenges

- Contraceptive pill/ condoms

- Heartburn relief

- Constipation relief

- Antifungal cream

- Antihistamine tablets

- Vitamin and mineral supplements such as vitamin c, vitamin d, calcium, iron, zinc

As your access to fresh fruit and vegetables and time outside in the sunshine may be limited, some vitamins and minerals may be beneficial. Read the packet instructions for how much to take and remember more is not always better!

Emergency Kit

Table 11 Family Emergency Kit

• Portable battery-operated AM/FM radio with extra batteries.
• Waterproof torch with extra batteries/ candles and waterproof matches.
• First aid kit and manual.
• Toilet paper and other sanitary items.
• Bottled drinking water for at least three days for each person (more if space is available).
• Canned or non-perishable food items for at least three days for each person. Can opener.
• Copies of important documents in a waterproof bag.
• Emergency contact phone numbers.
• Spare cash.
• Medications.

- Special items for babies, elderly or people with disabilities.

- Mobile/cell phone and charger.

- Spare house and car keys.

- Pet food and other needs.

- Cooking and eating gear/utensils.

- Small portable gas stove or alternative cooking device.

- Pot for boiling water plus water purification means.

- Pocket/utility knife.

- Change of clothing for everyone including gloves, hats enclosed shoes.

- Face mask/respirator.

- whistle.

- Spare glasses/contact lenses

- Light/glow sticks.

Store your emergency items in a sealable plastic container or weatherproof bag. If you do not have enough space in your container/bag, make a note of where other items can be found quickly.

Check and update the contents of your emergency kit every 12 months.

Attach your name and phone number to the bag.

Add a reminder tag to grab any prescription medication for family members to add to your pack.

Food Supply List

Tinned Food

Tinned vegetables e.g., corn, peas, beans, carrots, tomatoes.

Tinned soup

Tinned ready meals

Tinned fish e.g., tuna, salmon, sardines

Tinned meats e.g., corned beef, chicken, and spam

Tinned fruits

Baby food

Tinned beans and legumes

Tinned spaghetti/pasta

Dried Packaged Foods

Cereals e.g., porridge/oats

Pasta (spaghetti, noodles, instant, egg noodles and rice noodles)

Rice

Instant Noodles

Dried pasta meals

Powdered milk and baby formula

Flour

Corn flour

Baking powder/bi-carb soda

Sugar (brown and white)

Yeast

Bread mix

Tea/coffee/hot chocolate/Milo

Nuts (e.g., cashews, almonds, peanuts both salted and unsalted).

Pancake mix

Tomato paste (this can be used as a substitute for tinned tomatoes)

Corn chips

Packet cake and muffin mixes

Muesli bars/ energy bars,

Peanut butter/honey/vegemite/hazelnut spread/jam etc.

Herbs and spices

If you have a good supply of stock, herbs spices and sauces you can make anything taste delicious!

Salt and pepper

Onion powder or granules

Garlic powder or granules

Cumin

Coriander

Paprika

Oregano

Thyme

Chilli powder or Cayenne pepper

Curry powder

Mustard powder

Beef, vegetable and chicken stock powder or stock cubes (1 cube or 1 tsp powder in 1 cup / 250 ml boiling water = 1 cup stock). Buy stock cubes and powder instead of stock in cartons as it is cheaper and more space efficient.

Sauces, oils etc

Tomato/ketchup

BBQ

Worcestershire

Soy

Oyster

Sweet chilli

Gravy

Mustard

Pickles

Mirin

Chinese cooking wine

Red wine vinegar and white vinegar

Olive/vegetable/coconut/sunflower/sesame oils

Perishables

TIP Make sure you check the use by dates on your perishables and freeze or use them before the expiry date.

Beef, lamb, pork, chicken and fish or vegan alternatives. (These can also be frozen to extend their use-by date).

Milk/soymilk/almond milk etc. (long life and powdered versions of these can be purchased)

Cheeses- parmesan, tasty, mozzarella etc. (grated parmesan and mozzarella/tasty chesses can be frozen in zip lock bags).

Cream/sour cream

Fruit and vegetables (cut into small chunks and freeze in zip lock bags).

Eggs (these will keep in the fridge for several months)

Juice (box juices last longer).

Yogurt

Cold meats e.g., ham, bacon, salami (these can be frozen in bits)

Vegetables

Buy a variety of vegetables from tinned, fresh, and frozen. You can also freeze your own using zip lock bags, these can then be used in cooking.

Vegetables that can be frozen:

capsicum/bell peppers

onions brown, white and red

garlic

ginger

carrot

celery

corn

pumpkin

squash

zucchini

cauliflower

broccoli / broccolini

spinach

kale

limes (remove skin first and cut into wedges)

lemons (remove skin first and cut into wedges)

spring onions

(See the chapter on how to freeze fruit and vegetables).

Vegetables that have a long shelf life:

Potatoes

Cabbage

Carrots

Sweet potato

Brussel sprouts

Beetroot

Parsnip

Cauliflower

Onions

Spring onions

Garlic

Ginger

Vegetables such as lettuce, baby spinach, cucumbers tomatoes and other leafy greens have a shorter shelf life and don't freeze well. Do not purchase too many of these.

Fruit

Extend the life of your fruit by keeping it in the fridge especially in hot weather.

Freeze chopped fruit in zip lock bags for use in smoothies, slushies, and cakes.

Fruit that freezes well includes
Berries (blueberries, raspberries, strawberries)

Bananas (skin removed)

Mango

Pineapple

Apples

Tinned fruit and dried fruit are also a good alternative to fresh fruit and can be used in cooking.

Freezer

Beef, lamb, pork, chicken, and fish

Vegetables

Fruit packs

Pizza or other ready meals

Bread/Rolls

Ready rolled pastry

Fresh vegetables such as capsicum/bell peppers, and onions can be chopped and frozen in zip lock bags for later use.

Fresh peeled bananas, blueberries, mango, and raspberries can be frozen in zip lock bags for later use.

Egg whites can be frozen and used in cooking.

<u>Water and liquids</u>

Bottled water. It is wise to have a supply of bottled water available in case tap water is unavailable or unsafe to drink.

Bottled juice.

Long life milk, Almond milk/soy milk etc.

Coconut water/juice/milk

Stock e.g., beef, chicken, vegetable. (Stock cubes can also be used)

Some soft drinks

Alcohol

Energy drinks

Sports drinks with added electrolytes

Cooking oil, olive, vegetable, coconut, peanut

Sanitary Supply list

Hand sanitizer (if it is available! Or make your own)

Soap/body wash/hand wash

Deodorant

Toothpaste and toothbrushes plus a few extras for guests

Mouth wash

Tampons/pads for each female household member. Or washable period underwear such as Modibody.

Shampoo and conditioner

Chapstick and body lotion

Hand cream – hand sanitiser can be very drying on your skin.

Wet wipes – great if you are unable to wash.

Tissues

Toilet paper (2-3 rolls per person per week)

Cotton wool balls and buds/Q-tips.

Baby Supply list

Baby nappies/diapers

Wipes

Nappy/diaper rash cream

Nappy liners

Disposable nappy/diaper bags

Baby powder

Baby shampoo

Body lotion

Baby oil

Baby soap

Teething gel

Spare clothes, hat, bib, booties etc

Blankets

A few toys

Other household products

Paper towels (these can be used for drying hands rather than hand towels)

Clothes detergent or bar of laundry soap

Cleaning products

Bleach/disinfectant

Dishwashing liquid/dishwasher tablets and powder

Aluminium foil and cling wrap, baking paper.

Garbage bags

Waterproof Matches

Candles

Waterproof Torches

Spare Batteries

Zip lock bags (good for freezing meals, fruit and vegetables and water).

Steel wool (you can start a fire for a wood burner if you don't have matches by rubbing the steel wool against a 9-volt battery.)

Petroleum Jelly

A supply of plastic or paper plates, cups and utensils. These can be useful when your water supply is becoming low and you don't want to use your supplies for washing plates etc.

Disinfectant wipes

Acknowledgments

How much water do you need? Centre of Disease Control
 https://www.cdc.gov

World Health Organisation
https://www.who.int/gpsc/5may/Guide_to_Local_Production.pdf

https://www.who.int/howmuchwaterisneededinemergencies

Purifying water during an emergency.
https://www.doh.wa.gov

How do water purification tablets work? Carolyn Graves 2020
 https://www.okeanostech.com

How to make an emergency water filter.
 https://www.H2Odistributers.com

Fire blankets and extinguishers.
https://www.dfes.wa.wa.gov.au/fire

Travelling during a bushfire

Bushfire Overview - Department of Fire and
Emergency Services (dfes.wa.gov.au)

Hypothermia
https://www.health.nsw.gov.au

Hyperthermia: too hot for your health.
https://www.nih.gov

Emergency Preparedness ad response.
https://www.bt.cdc.gov/radiation/contamination

Surviving a bushfire when it's too late to leave.
https://www.rac.com.au/home-life/info/bushfire-
survive

Earthquake Safety Information Sheet.
https://www.defs.wa.gov/safteyinformation/earth
quakes

Cyclone, hurricane, typhoon. What's the difference?
https://www.bbc.news

Hurricanes and Tropical cyclones.
https://www.weather.gov

Tsunami
https://www.departmentofifreandemergencyservic
es/safetyinformation

What to do in a Tsunami.
https://www.ses.vic.gov.au/get-eady/tsunamisafe/what-to-do-in-a-tsunami

How to prepare for a flood.

https://www.bom.gov.au/hydro/floods

How to perform CPR.

https://www.healthdirect.gov.au/how-to-perform-cpr

First Aid

St John's Ambulance First Aid Manual 2020

7 tips for storing food in Mylar bags.

https://www.alloutdoor.com

Saffir-Simpson Hurricane Scale.

Https://www.ready.gov/america/beinformed/hurricanes

Tornado Safety. Roger Edwards.

https://www.spc.noaa.gov

First aid for shock

https://www.healthywa.wa.giv.au

The good living guide to Natural and herbal remedies
Katolen Yardley (2016).

Pets and Other Animals
https://www.defs.wa.gov.au

About the Author

Suzanne was born in Perth Western Australia and as a young adult grew up in the small country town of Tom Price situated in the outback of Australia. Her current home is in Perth with her husband and two daughters.

Suzanne has a Bachelor of Science Degree, and her hobbies include running, gardening, photography and prepping. Her interest in prepping began after the 2009 Black Saturday bushfires in Australia. After seeing how quickly people's lives could be disrupted by a disaster, she wanted to ensure her family was prepared.

She has published four novels including the award-winning YA survival series *Seventeen* set in the harsh

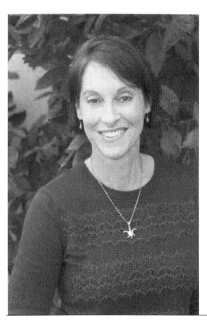

Australian outback. *Seventeen* was awarded best Sci-Fi/Horror for an eBook by the New Apple literary awards and also received a bronze medal from Readers' Favorite International writers' competition.

In 2020 her middle grade fiction novel *The Pirate Princess and the Golden Locket* was awarded both a bronze medal and a Book Excellence Award in Pre-Teen Literature.

Suzanne is a member of the Society of Children's Book Writers and Illustrators, Travel Writers Association, Australian Society of Authors, and the Australian Science Fiction Society.

You can follow Suzanne through her social media accounts.

www.Suzanneloweauthor.com

www.twitter.com/@Suzanne_Lowe_
www.instagram.com/suzannelowe.author/
www.facebook.com/suzanneloweauthor/

Other Books by the Author

Seventeen

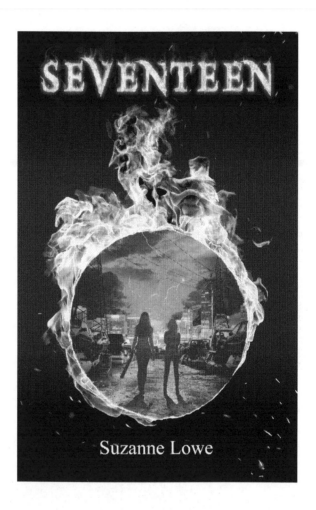

**Winner of the New Apple YA horror/Sci-Fi award
Bronze Medal Winner- Readers Favorite**

Imagine a world where everything you grew up with is gone. No adults, no internet, no rules. Could you survive?

The world is facing the deadliest virus ever known.

When the KV17 virus kills everyone above the age of seventeen, life becomes a battle of survival for the children left behind. Seeking to escape the escalating violence in the city, two sisters, Lexi and Hadley flee to the Australian outback. Finding sanctuary in the small town of Jasper's Bay, they soon realise it is far from safe, as a gang of lawless teenagers terrorise the town.

Caught in a bitter feud leading to betrayal, deceit and murder, the girls must quickly uncover who their enemies are, and who they can trust. In a world drastically changed from everything they once knew; can the sisters and children of Jasper's Bay learn to adapt? Can they maintain control of their town, and protect it from those who would destroy it?

www.suzanneloweauthor.com

www.silvergumpublishing.com

Rage

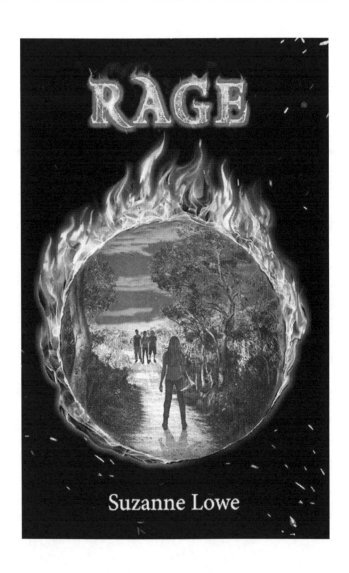

"Some acts can never be forgiven."

The story of sisters Lexi and Hadley continues in book two of the *Seventeen Series.*

With the KV17 virus now in its mutated form not even the children are safe. Can Lexi and her friends survive this new threat? An exciting survival story set in the Australian outback.

www.suzanneloweauthor.com
www.silvergumpublishing.com

The Pirate Princess and The Golden Locket

Book one in the *Pirate Princess* Series.

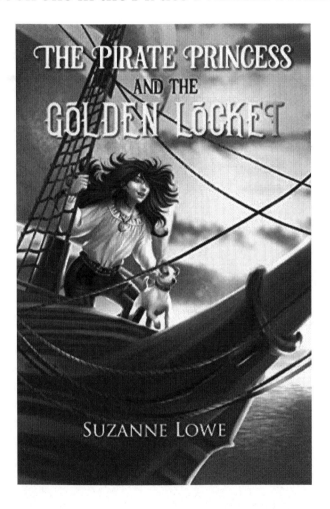

The first thrilling tale of adventure, friendship and mystery in the Pirate Princess series.

The Pirate Princess and the Golden Locket is an exciting adventure story for 6-11-year-old children.

Meet Lotty, the brave young orphan whose life is suddenly about to change forever.

When on her twelfth birthday, Lotty is unexpectantly cast out from the Sevenoaks Home for Children, she befriends a cheeky little dog called Mr. Jacks. Her life soon becomes an exciting adventure as together they encounter lazy pirates, hidden treasure and uncover the mystery of Lotty's golden locket!

The Pirate Princess and the Golden Locket is a story full of loveable characters, swashbuckling adventures and ruthless pirates!

www.suzanneloweauthor.com
www.silvergumpublishing.com

The Pirate Princess and The Sirens' Song

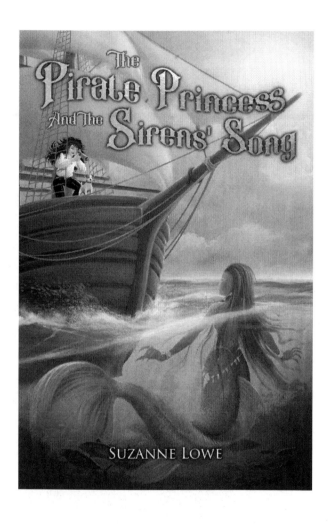

Lotty' and Mr Jacks adventures continue in this exciting new book *The Pirate Princess and the Sirens' Song.*

Can Lotty find what the Sirens most desire and save the pirates or will they be trapped on the mysterious island forever?

www.suzanneloweauthor.com
www.silvergumpublishing.com

Made in the USA
Las Vegas, NV
04 April 2021